Reinventing Depression

Reinventing Depression

A History of the Treatment of Depression in Primary Care, 1940–2004

CHRISTOPHER M. CALLAHAN, M.D.
Indiana University School of Medicine

GERMAN E. BERRIOS, M.D.
University of Cambridge

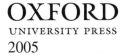

UNIVERSITY PRESS
2005

OXFORD

UNIVERSITY PRESS

Oxford   New York
Auckland   Bangkok   Buenos Aires   Cape Town   Chennai
Dar es Salaam   Delhi   Hong Kong   Istanbul   Karachi   Kolkata
Kuala Lumpur   Madrid   Melbourne   Mexico City   Mumbai   Nairobi
São Paulo   Shanghai   Taipei   Tokyo   Toronto

Published by Oxford University Press, Inc.
198 Madison Avenue, New York, New York 10016
www.oup.com

Oxford is a registered trademark of Oxford University Press

Library of Congress Cataloging-in-Publication Data
Callahan, Christopher M.
Reinventing depression : a history of the treatment of depression in primary care,
1940–2004 / Christopher M. Callahan, German E. Berrios.
p. ; cm.
Includes bibliographical references and index.
ISBN 0-19-516523-3
1. Depression, Mental—Treatment—Great Britain—History—20th century.   2. Depression,
Mental—Treatment—United States—History—20th century.   3. Primary care
(Medicine)—Great Britain—History—20th century.   4. Primary care (Medicine)—United
States—History—20th century.   I. Berrios, G. E.   II. Title.
[DNLM: 1. Depressive Disorder—therapy.   2. History of Medicine, 20th Cent.   3. Primary
Health Care—methods.   WM 171 C156r 2004]
RC537.C25 2004
616.85'27—dc22   2004047790

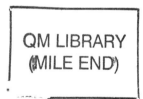
9   8   7   6   5   4   3   2   1

Printed in the United States of America
on acid-free paper

For Missy, Bluey, and Birdy—
thanks for the adventure

Preface

Each year, the United States and the United Kingdom spend billions to treat depression. Despite these costs, depression remains one of the most underrecognized, undertreated, and disabling conditions in both countries. At the same time, depression is one of the most common reasons that people seek care from generalist physicians; these primary-care doctors treat most patients suffering from depression. Unfortunately, advances in medical science have not led to a decline in depression in either country.

While new strategies for diagnosing and treating depression have improved millions of people's lives, there is little evidence that the overall societal burden of depression has decreased. In contrast, the application of public health techniques, coupled with antibiotic medications, led to a dramatic decline in morbidity and mortality from infectious diseases in industrialized countries in the twentieth century. Along the same lines, early interventions for the risk factors associated with cardiovascular disease precipitated a decline in morbidity and mortality from heart attack and stroke. Why have we not seen a similar decline in morbidity and mortality from depression? Most experts point to a gap between what psychiatrists *know* and what primary-care doctors *do* to explain untreated depression. We argue, however, that untreated depression is caused by a lack of attention to a public health perspective that would emphasize the role of individual and community responsibility.

The central premise of this book is that depression and the current treatment models associated with it are so narrowly defined that only a limited number of patients will seek and benefit from care. Current etiologic models that explain how depression progresses underestimate the roles of society and culture in causing depression and overemphasize biological aspects. These models are too deterministic and fail to reveal how much they have changed in the past 50 years.

This book emphasizes how the definition of depression has changed over time. The definition of depression which identifies it as an illness that explains emotional suffering, opens a pathway for seeking medical help, and offers a model for providing care is an invention that is less than a quarter-century old. In the 1950s, organized medicine had given emotional suffering other labels, ascribed other causes to it, and provided different treatments, which had replaced those from earlier in the century. The invention and reinvention not only changed medical terms and treatments but also changed how society views people with emotional symptoms, defines who is sick, and determines who should seek and receive care. Each reinvention also influences public decisions regarding who should pay for and who should benefit from providing care. The definition and treatment of depression are important inventions of science and society that enable us to care for people in need. The title of this book emphasizes that the invention is not static. It has changed frequently and will continue to change.

While we refer most often to "depression," the terminology of emotional disorders has been fluid, and thus our scope includes a broad array of affective or mood disorders. For example, much of the early work in this field dealt with emotional symptoms or diagnoses such as "neurosis" rather than with explicit psychiatric diagnoses as currently defined. In retelling this story, we adopt the language of each period that was used to label emotional disorders (Berrios and Porter 1995). These terms are not synonyms for "depression." It is also important to recognize that labels have consequences: The language of emotional disorders carries significant meanings and influences the behavior of patients, providers, and policy makers (Berrios 1985).

When referring to primary care, we use the following terms interchangeably: primary care, general practice, general health care, general medicine settings, general medical care, family practice, and family medicine. We also use the terms general practitioner, primary-care physician, family physician, and generalist to denote the physician working in the primary-care environment. While these terms are not necessarily interchangeable, their overlap in meaning and practice is so substantial that we treat the terms as synonyms in this book. In addition, public health experts often refer to primary care as first-contact health care. The World Health Organization (1978) defines primary health care as:

Essential health care, based on practical, scientifically sound, socially acceptable methods and technology, made universally accessible to individuals and families in the community, through their full participation and at a cost the community and the country can afford. It forms an integral part of both the country's health system, of which it is the central function and main focus, and of the overall social and economic development of the community.

To tell the broader story of depression, it is important to describe the story of scientific discoveries within psychiatry. We are arguing, however, that since World War I and especially since World War II, the story of primary care rivals psychiatry's importance in the care of depression. The current labels, causes, and treatments for depression are not the end of this process—they are simply the latest chapter. We can better understand the strengths and weaknesses of the latest reinvention by taking a historical perspective that includes changes in both science and society. Central to this historical perspective is the story of primary-care medicine.

Primary-care doctors provide most of the care for patients with depression. Experts do not debate this fact, yet the current, narrow approach to depression fails to take advantage of primary care's potential strengths. Chief among these strengths are the primary-care doctor's ability to manage the patient's entire constellation of medical conditions, to understand the broad context of the patient's emotional symptoms, and to enlist the patient and the community in prevention and treatment. Unfortunately, primary care does not effectively use this potential. Also, the primary-care profession and society remain ambivalent about expanding primary care's role to include the health of communities. This ambivalence stems from our discomfort in the ambiguous zone between public health mandates and personal liberty.

This book tells the still-unfolding story of why we seek and how we receive care for emotional disorders and how both science and society influence our decisions. We will not see progress in the care of depression until we understand where we are and how we got here. Ideas about the causes and treatments of depression have changed dramatically over the past half-century. Social viewpoints and world events have at least as great a role as scientific discovery has in precipitating these changes. Primary-care medicine is at the focal point of care for depression. Thus, the reinvention of depression plays out on the stage of primary care, and changes on this stage influence the reinvention at least as much as discoveries in psychiatry do.

Most books about the history of depression focus only on developments in psychiatry or psychopharmacology, failing to recognize the influential role of primary care. This narrower perspective also fails to integrate the advances in psychiatry or psychopharmacology with other medical discoveries and changes in the spectrum of human illness, and it ignores society's important role in modulating help-seeking behaviors for problems like depression. We embrace these complexities and thus present a more complete picture of the reinvention of depression.

Our challenge in organizing this book comes not from a lack of information but from how to best communicate the intertwined histories in a readable fashion. In telling this story, we considered organizing the book as a strict chronology of events. That approach, however, would have exaggerated discrete events and distorted the incremental, interrelated, and serendipitous nature of the reinvention. To capture the broader perspective, we decided to focus on a series of six interconnected stories, each unfolding over the past 50 years. We start with a core thread and then successively weave in five more threads.

Six Interconnected Stories Describing the Reinvention of Depression Over the Past Half Century

1. How did primary-care patients seek help and how did doctors provide treatment for emotional symptoms during the past half century?
2. How has the primary-care environment changed and which social and scientific factors were important in causing these changes?
3. How did new drugs help change the nature of illness cared for by primary-care doctors and how did this change society's expectations for medical care?
4. How was psychiatry's transformed after World War II through the major discoveries in psychopharmacology?
5. How did primary care physicians develop a nonspecific approach to emotional disorders in primary care and what was the role of the pharmaceutical industry?
6. How have psychiatrists attempted to improve the specificity and effectiveness of treatment for depression in primary care?

The core thread is the story of how primary-care patients sought help and how doctors have provided treatment for emotional symptoms during the past half century. The second thread describes how the primary-care environment changed and which social and scientific factors were important in causing these changes. The third thread tells how new drugs helped change the nature of illness cared for by primary-care doctors and how this changed society's expectations for medical care, which, in turn, affected the role of primary-care doctors. These first three stories paint the picture of primary care because it is on this canvas that most people receive health care for depression.

After describing primary care, we take a step back in time to tell the fourth story about psychiatry's transformation after World War II and the major discoveries in psychopharmacology. This fourth thread is about patients with psychiatric conditions who receive care from specialty psychiatry rather than primary care (schizophrenia, for example). This is an important story because the disease-specific treatment model for these psychiatric disorders will eventually collide with the nonspecific treatment model for emotional disorders that are typical of primary care, which is the main theme of the fifth thread. This fifth thread also addresses the important role of the pharmaceutical industry, as opposed to psychiatry, in offering treatments for emotional disorders in primary care before 1975. It is only in the last quarter of the twentieth century that psychiatry came to discover this new world of psychiatric morbidity in primary care. The sixth and final thread traces psychiatrists' efforts to improve the specificity and effectiveness of treatment for depression in primary care and how they attempted to disseminate this new model. Through these six intertwined stories, we outline the strengths and limits of the latest reinvention of depression.

Understanding these strengths and limitations helps us see why depression's burden on the community has not decreased. The current treatment model, which was developed by specialty psychiatry and accepted by primary care, reinforces the idea that we can treat depression in a relatively narrow, mainly biological way. This limited model fails to realize primary care's full potential. In most respects, primary-care doctors have either delegated or abdicated their leadership role in treating people with emotional disorders to psychiatric specialists, other health-care professionals, researchers, industry, and policy makers. Primary-care doctors limit their participation in research, practice redesign, and policy on emotional disorders. This is not a fault of psychiatry or the industry—rather, it points to a failure of primary care leadership.

The reinvention of depression in the past half-century indicates real progress. Yet if we do not expose the current model's assumptions, conventions, and limits, continued progress will be stalled. Primary-care doctors need not and should not receive treatment guidelines passively. Instead, they must embrace their central role in the care of patients with emotional disorders and in the continual reinvention of depression. Taking this role inevitably will lead general physicians to consider the multiple determinants of emotional health that currently remain outside the range of primary care, such as the social and physical environment, education, and economic opportunity, among others.

This expanding role for primary care will compel society to weigh the advantages and disadvantages of a primary-care system that increasingly concerns itself with community health. Primary care and society already struggle with these issues in such areas as lifestyle behaviors and preventive measures for cardiovascular disease, for example. Reinventing depression, however, may demand that primary care reach even further into difficult social problems. Depression may help reinvent primary care by pushing these boundaries. For this reason, we wrote this book not just for health services researchers and mental health specialists but for the larger community of providers, patients, and advocates who seek to improve the lives of people with depression through prevention and treatment.

Indianapolis, Indiana   C.C.
Cambridge, United Kingdom   G. B.

Acknowledgments

We would like to acknowledge the important editorial contributions of Jeffrey W. House and Donna Maurer, Ph.D. Dr. Callahan was supported by a Paul B. Beeson Physician Faculty Scholars in Aging Research Award administered by the American Federation for Aging Research and by grants from the John A. Hartford Foundation, Inc. and the National Institute on Aging [K07 AG00868]. Callahan also is supported through the Cornelius and Yvonne Pettinga Chair in Aging Research and the Regenstrief Institute, Inc. The authors collaborated on this work during a year of sabbatical while Callahan was a visiting scholar in the history and psychopathology research program in the department of psychiatry at Cambridge University working under the mentorship of Dr. Berrios.

Contents

Part III   Lessons Learned and Moving Forward

Reinventing Depression

Part I

THE CARE OF EMOTIONAL
DISORDERS IN PRIMARY CARE

1

WHY DEPRESSION?

Depression is a killer. It kills dreams, marriages, and people. As the history of reinventing depression unfolds, and as we recount the serendipitous discoveries and cultural conventions surrounding this illness, we do not wish to minimize the suffering that depression causes. No part of this history suggests that depression and emotional problems are not important public health concerns. To highlight the importance of depression from the very outset of this book, we first review recent information about both its global and its personal impact. We then present a general model for the causes of depression and outline the current treatment model for depression in primary care. The goal of this chapter, therefore, is to summarize the experience of depression in our communities.

The Burden of Depression

The World Health Organization estimates that 450 million people worldwide suffer from a mental illness and that one in four people will suffer from mental illness at some point in their lives (see Box, next page). Mental illness may account for as much as one-third of all disability (Murray and Lopez 1996; World Health Organization 2001). It is estimated that depressive disorders afflict 121 million people globally and account for 10% of all people seeking care from generalist physicians. Among patients with a major depressive disorder, as many as 15%

Current Treatment Model for Depression

According to the World Health Organization (WHO), neuropsychiatric disorders account for 31% of the disability in the world, affecting rich and poor nations and individuals alike. Because people do not get the care they need, mental and neurological disorders impose various costs on individuals, households, employers, and society as a whole, ranging from the cost of care to the cost of lost productivity.

The magnitude of the mental health burden is not matched by the size and effectiveness of the response it receives. Currently, over one-third of countries assign less than 1% of their total health budgets to mental health, and another one-third devote just 1% of their budgets to it. The current treatment model includes these 10 features, as recommended by the WHO:

1. Provide treatment in primary care
2. Make psychotropic medicines available
3. Provide care in the community
4. Educate the public
5. Involve communities, families, and consumers
6. Establish national policies, programs, and legislation
7. Develop human resources
8. Link with other sectors
9. Monitor community mental health
10. Support more research

Source: World Health Organization. *World Health Report 2001—Mental Health: New Understanding, New Hope.* Geneva: World Health Organization, 2001.

may eventually die by suicide (Sainsbury 1986). Suicide is one of the top 10 leading causes of death in the United States and the United Kingdom, causing 1.6% of deaths worldwide. One million people kill themselves each year (World Health Organization 2001), and depression is the primary disorder in 60% of these cases.

Depression causes both emotional and physical disability. In economically developed regions of the world, it is second only to ischemic heart disease as the leading cause of disability (Murray and Lopez 1996). In developed countries, depression is the leading cause of disability among people ages 15–44 (Murray and Lopez 1996). Self-inflicted injuries and suicide, often associated with depressive illness, also contribute to the burden of disability. Clearly, depression represents an enormous source of suffering across the globe.

Often viewed simply as a mental illness, depression causes a decline in physical performance. Patients with depression report such physical symptoms as a lack of energy, fatigue, weakness, slowed movements, agitation, insomnia, difficulty concentrating, and pain. The physical pain experienced by some patients with depression is as real and incapacitating as the pain associated with medical conditions. Indeed, the pain often mimics that caused by common medical conditions and thereby clouds the diagnosis. The extent of the physical disability can be as severe as, or more severe than, such common, chronic medical conditions as heart disease, diabetes, and arthritis (Wells et al. 1989). Depression also compounds the effects of chronic medical conditions. Emotional disorders lead to loss of work productivity, including days of missed work and days confined to bed (Broadhead et al. 1990). One reason for highlighting the physical effects of depression is to communicate the reality of an illness that often seems abstract. The feeling that people with depression simply need to pick themselves up by their own bootstraps endures as a prejudice. Because a depressed person's family and friends cannot see the injury and may not be able to empathize by calling on their own experience, the illness may not seem real. Even worse, people *may* call on their own experience with minor emotional upheavals and celebrate their strength in overcoming blue moods, rather than empathize with the person suffering from depression.

Because the wounds of depression remain veiled, many have struggled to communicate their pain in a manner comprehensible to those who have not experienced it. William Styron (1990), the author of *The Confessions of Nat Turner* and *Sophie's Choice*, described it this way:

What I had begun to discover is that, mysteriously and in ways that are totally remote from normal experience, the gray drizzle of horror induced by depression takes on the quality of physical pain. But it is not an immediately identifiable pain, like that of a broken limb. It may be more accurate to say that despair, owing to some evil trick played upon the sick brain by the inhabiting psyche, comes to resemble the diabolical discomfort of being imprisoned in a fiercely overheated room. And because no breeze stirs this cauldron, because there is no escape from this smothering confinement, it is entirely natural that the victim begins to think ceaselessly of oblivion.

The blurred boundaries between a normal, passing emotion and an intractable, devastating disease, coupled with the elusive nature of mental illness, help explain centuries of misunderstanding and mistreatment. Mental health advocates' strategy to frame the etiology of emotional disorders in a biomedical and physical context, however, has had important and unanticipated ramifications. This strategy influenced not only how patients, policy makers, and the public view the illness but also how physicians approach treatment and how scientists conduct research. Distinguishing between depression "the disease," depression "the symptom," and depression "the experience" is one of the most difficult problems facing physicians and patients, and we often get it wrong.

Etiologic Models of Affective Disorders

Over the past 50 years, scientists have proposed multiple biological explanations for the cause of depression and the response to antidepressant treatments. Despite this work, there is no agreement on a final, common, biological pathway. In a recent review, a consortium of experts on the biology of depression, including representatives from the National Institute of Mental Health, concluded: "We have not identified the genetic and neurobiological mechanisms underlying depression and mania, nor do we understand the mechanisms by which nongenetic factors influence these disorders" (Nestler et al. 2002). Without such specificity, researchers rely instead on models that incorporate the many broad determinants of emotional disorders. There are numerous etiologic models for affective disorders in general and depressive disorders in particular. These models attempt to explain why some people get depression and others do not. Nearly all of them suggest an interaction between predisposition (genes) and environment (stressors). The environmental causes run the gamut from psychosocial stressors of every variety to physical illness, specific toxins, exposures, and developmental aberrations. The model of affective disorders presented in Figure 1–1 was adapted from several different sources (Lewis 1953; Akiskal and McKinney 1975; Billings and Moos 1982; Friedland and McColl 1992; Risch 1997; Honig and van Praag 1997; Nuki 1999; Teasdale 1999). The term "affective disorders" refers to a variety of emotional disorders, including depression, manic depression, and anxiety.

This etiologic model highlights the potential for both biological and psychosocial causes to initiate a cascade of physiologic and behavioral reactions that lead to depression. It suggests that everyone is at risk for depression if exposed to a critical level of stressors. An individual's personal and environmental coping capacity moderates his or her reaction to the abnormal physiology or environment. Some individuals will be able to call on these capacities to cope and adapt to the adverse conditions, while others will not. Recognizing that all individuals experience physiologic or environmental stress, Aubrey Lewis (1953) defined mental health as "a state of perfect equipoise in an unstable environment." Lewis was among the early leaders in academic psychiatry after World War II. Individuals may judge differently than their family, physicians, or community whether their responses to the stress have been successful and healthy. In Figure 1–1, arrows lead back from the box labeled "affective disorder" to the boxes labeled "abnormal nervous system function" and "abnormal stress." This suggests that depression itself causes either abnormality, thus perpetuating the illness even after the initial cause is removed. Some authors suggest that behavioral, cellular, or subcellular responses may result in a self-perpetuating depressive illness (Risch 1997).

Mental health experts currently recognize several specific risk factors for depression. These include prior episodes of depression, family history of depressive disorder, prior suicide attempts, female gender, age of onset under 40, postpartum

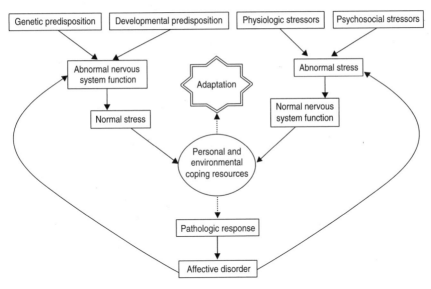

FIGURE 1–1. Etiologic model of affective disorders.

period, medical comorbidity, lack of social support, stressful life events, and current substance abuse. Medications used to treat other disorders also have been associated with increased risk for depression (Depression Guideline Panel 1993).

Despite the consensus agreement that we do not understand the genetic and neurobiological mechanisms of depression (Nestler et al. 2002), mental health leaders and advocates have continued to espouse a biological model of depression that focuses on neurotransmitters. In this model, depression is depicted as a disruption of normal brain neurochemistry. Neurotransmitters, of which there are many types, are the brain's messengers and operate in the spaces between adjacent brain cells by transmitting signals from cell to cell. Some of these neurotransmitters are believed to play a central role in the pathology of depression. This neurotransmitter model was developed nearly simultaneously with the development of the first effective antidepressant medications, and the model has endured despite a lack of supporting scientific evidence. At minimum, this model conveys an oversimplification of how antidepressant drugs work.

The neurotransmitter model of depression endures for at least three reasons. First, it provides a compelling explanation for why antidepressant medications are an effective treatment for depression, and it has proved to be an effective model to guide the development of new drug treatments for depression. Second, it provides a plausible final common biological pathway for all of the many reasons why a person might become depressed. Third, it offers a very powerful message in mental health advocacy. After centuries of blaming mental health on demons and personal weakness, society now has a biological model to explain depression. This model is every bit as compelling as biological models explaining heart disease. The neurotransmitter model guides not only research, but also the content of physician–patient interactions about the causes and treatment of depression.

Diagnosing and Treating Depression

Several authoritative panels have published updated guidelines on depression's diagnosis and treatment, with many of these guidelines focusing specifically on primary care as the site for treating depression (Depression Guideline Panel 1993; Katz and Alexopoulos 1996; Ballenger et al. 1999; WHO Collaborating Centre for Mental Health Research and Training 2000). In general, the expert panels recommend a clinical approach that can be summarized as follows. Providers should:

1. Recognize the presenting symptoms of depression and its causes.
2. Make an explicit diagnosis of depression.
3. Educate the patient and family, and stress that depression is treatable.
4. Engage the patient and family in choosing treatment.
5. Assess patients' progress regularly.

Current treatment recommendations imply that depression is a specific biomedical disease, and the practical realities of caring for patients in primary care increase the focus on drug therapy. Most current treatment choices, and, more important, most health-care systems, cannot intervene on precipitating causes of depression (for example, economic or social stressors). Counseling, psychotherapy, and access to community agencies may enhance patients' capacity to cope with these stressors, but providers typically cannot simply remove them. Although some experts have recommended a more community-based approach, the current treatment model rests on a patient–physician interaction in a health-care setting. Many patients who need treatment for affective disorders never seek care for their emotional distress. Current treatment models do not provide guidance on how to reach people outside the health-care system or those within the system who do not seek care for their emotional problems.

Description of the Current Treatment Model

Typically, the treatment of depression begins with a patient visiting a health-care provider and reporting symptoms that suggest a mood disorder. These symptoms might be direct reports of sadness or depression, but often the emotional symptoms are hidden behind a report of physical complaints such as fatigue. The diagnosis of a treatable depression requires that the patient report depressed mood or loss of interest or pleasure for most of the time for two or more weeks. In addition, the diagnosis requires the presence of at least four of the following eight symptoms: difficulty with sleep, loss of interest of pleasure, guilt, loss of energy, diminished concentration, increased or decreased appetite, observed psychomotor agitation or retardation, or thoughts of suicide. If the patient meets these criteria, the doctor diagnoses a major depressive disorder. This distinguishes the patient's reporting symptoms from more minor fluctuations in mood and from other medical causes of the common symptoms. After making a specific diagnosis, the physician then can chose a therapy specific for that diagnosis.

Once the patient has been diagnosed, the doctor explains the diagnosis and prognosis and educates the patient about available treatments, including their risks, benefits, costs, availability, and expected success rate. The patient (and perhaps his or her family members) then makes an informed choice regarding which treatment to pursue. The two most common treatments available in primary care are psychotherapy and antidepressant medications. By far, the most commonly prescribed treatment is antidepressant medication. This occurs due to physician and patient factors, as well as the availability and acceptability of other therapies. Recent research has demonstrated that diagnosis and treatment initiation are just the beginning of effective treatment for depression. Providers and health-care systems also must help the patient adhere to the therapy, monitor progress over time, adjust therapy as needed, and provide care until the symptoms completly resolve.

Effectiveness of the Current Treatment Model

Although the treatment model described above rests on a foundation of a specific physician diagnosis based on the presence of a specific constellation of symptoms, primary-care physicians often use a nonspecific approach. In other words, antidepressant drugs are specific treatments for a specific diagnosis, but these drugs, and other psychoactive agents, are often used to treat nonspecific symptoms that do not meet the criteria for a specific diagnosis. This lack of specificity in diagnosis and treatment undermines the effectiveness of the current treatment model. In other words, many people who might benefit from treatment are not receiving treatment, and many people who cannot benefit from treatment are receiving treatment.

The extent of this problem is worldwide and was dramatically revealed by a 1990 study conducted by the World Health Organization (WHO) examining the effectiveness of the current treatment model. The purpose of this study was to "investigate the frequency, form, recognition, management, course and outcome of psychological disorders encountered in general health settings." The study was carried out at 15 general medicine clinics in 15 different countries, including the United Kingdom and the United States (Ustun and Sartorius 1995). Across all the centers, 24% of the study participants had a current mental disorder, 9% had significant symptoms but not sufficient to constitute a mental disorder, 31% reported at least some psychological symptoms, and 36% were well. Even though the psychiatrists used the same diagnostic criteria across all 15 sites, the rates of mental illness ranged from a low of 7.3% to a high of 52.5% at different sites. The researchers speculated that, rather than reflecting a true difference in the rates of illness, much of this variation was due to differences in sociodemographics, help-seeking behavior, and study participation rates. Depression was the most common diagnosis (10.4%), followed by anxiety (7.9%). In all the centers, patients with mental disorders tended to present with physical symptoms and underreport their emotional symptoms. Primary-care physicians rated their patients with psychiatric diagnoses as more physically ill and having more chronic conditions, greater disability, and poorer health. Patients with a psychiatric disorder reported an average of six days of disability each month.

In the WHO study, there was only modest agreement between the primary-care physicians' diagnoses of mental illness and the diagnostic criteria used by the research team. Across all the centers, the researchers found that 32.5% of patients met diagnostic criteria for psychiatric illness, while the primary-care physicians diagnosed only 24.2%. More important, the diagnoses of researchers and primary-care physicians matched in only 13.3% of the cases. This represents a substantial disagreement among the researchers and practitioners regarding which patients need specific treatment. Primary-care physicians reported that they treated 77.8% of the people who they diagnosed with a mental illness. Their choice of treatments included counseling (52.9%), sedative medications (26.3%), and antidepressant medications (15%). In all the centers, doctors chose the same types of treatment, whether or not they diagnosed depression, anxiety, or somatoform disorder (a condition in which the patient experiences emotional distress as physical symptoms). Because nearly all authoritative panels over the past 20 years have espoused specific treatments for depressive illness, this finding surprised the investigators. Although this study is not necessarily representative of the care provided for those with depression throughout the United States and the United Kingdom, a wealth of health-services research completed during the past few decades supports these findings. Primary-care physicians prescribe nonspecific drugs to treat their patients' nonspecific emotional symptoms. Is this due simply to a gap between what the experts know and how the doctors practice, or does this point to an important limitation in the treatment model?

A study by Schulberg and colleagues (1996) exemplifies the potential and the limitations of the current treatment guidelines for depression in primary care. In this study, approximately two-thirds of primary-care patients who received standard-of-care treatment for depression experienced a significant improvement in their symptoms. One-third of the patients did not improve, although perhaps half of them might have responded to more aggressive treatment in a psychiatry clinic. Thus, as many as 80% of patients who receive therapy for depression could experience at least a short-term improvement in their symptoms. Mental health advocates typically use this 80% figure as a benchmark to highlight the potential success of the current treatment model if it were applied appropriately.

We highlight three caveats about these reported success rates. First, a study's experimental conditions may partially explain higher recovery rates. For example, research personnel typically encourage adherence to treatment and closely monitor patients' progress. Second, even under experimental conditions, the 80% response rate only applies to patients who complete an adequate course of therapy. Unfortunately, 40% to 60% of patients who begin treatment for depression do not complete their course of therapy, and thus they are not included in the study sample. These low rates of adherence are true for patients who are prescribed newer antidepressant drugs, as well as psychotherapy. Third, patients with depression complicated by other serious medical or psychiatric disorders do not respond to treatment well. In naturalistic studies of "usual care" in primary-care settings, treated patients' response rates are as low as 10% to 30% (Ormel and van den Brink 1993; Schulberg et al. 1997; Thase 1999; Cole et al. 1999).

In a review of the course and outcome of depression, Duggan (1997) reported that

even with the most generous estimates, only two-thirds of those treated with either psychological or physical treatments can expect to have a prompt response to treatment and a further 15% will fail to recover at all from the episode and become chronic. Second, among the successful responders, at least a third will have another relapse while in remission and hence fail to recover. Third, for those who recover, another episode is likely in 75% of the cases with the same cycle being repeated.

Duggan estimated that for every 100 patients treated with an adequate course of therapy for depression,

66 can expect to respond to treatment and 10–15 will remain chronic. Of the 66 responders, 22 will have a relapse during the phase of remission. Of the 44 who recover, 33 can expect a recurrence with the cycle being repeated. According to these figures, only 11% can expect to progress to recovery and remain well without further episodes.

In addition to these 100 patients receiving an adequate course of therapy, at least another 100 patients seen in primary care and diagnosed with depression will not receive adequate therapy. Still another 100 patients will not seek care or, if they seek care, will remain undiagnosed and receive no treatment. Epidemiologists have estimated that as many as half the people with emotional disorders who could benefit from treatment never seek care for their illnesses (Department of Health and Human Services 1999). For many patients seeking care for depression, the current treatment model is effective, but for many others, the model is simply inadequate.

The current model seems to have resulted in a significant, societal problem: Only about half the people with emotional symptoms seek care from a doctor. Does this mean they do not need care or that we need better outreach? For patients who do seek care, the question remains, "What is the origin of my distress and who is able to help me?" Not all will view medical treatment as the source of care. For those who do seek medical care for emotional symptoms, general practitioners still struggle to determine which patients should receive what treatment. For policy makers, the questions are, "How do we define mental health services needs, how do we provide for these needs, and how do we assess the outcomes of care?" (Verhaak 1995). Thus, in assessing the strengths and limitations of the current treatment model, opinions range from an optimistic "look how far the field has come" to a pessimistic "look how far we need to go."

Summary

A large volume of medical literature documents three important findings about depression. These three findings provide a solid answer to the question "Why does depression matter?" First, depression is common and disabling. Second, etiologic models of depression suggest that the environment and coping capacity, among other determinants, are at least as important as genetics and neurochemistry in explaining the causes of depression. Yet the current treatment model overemphasizes the biological origins of the disorder. Third, epidemiologic studies and clinical trials of primary-care patients demonstrate the clear limitations of the current model. Using this approach may not reach at least half of the people who could benefit from care.

We have educated an entire generation of physicians, patients, and potential patients with an overly deterministic model that suggests that an imbalance of brain chemicals causes depression. Correcting that hypothetical imbalance cures depression. The consumers in this generation view this model as long-standing and well-established. For some time, experts in psychiatry and public health have argued that the continued burden of depression stems from a poor application of this model in primary care, where most patients receive care for depression. In this book, we build the argument that the *limited applicability* of the treatment model is at least as important as its *limited application* in explaining the continued burden of depression.

To build this argument effectively, we must paint a broader picture of the primary-care practice setting and how primary-care patients seek care for emotional disturbances. We also need to document how the setting and the patients have changed over time. We seek to tell a more complete story of how changes independent of developments in psychiatry shape treatment for emotional disorders in primary care. In the next chapter, the story begins with how primary-care physicians treated patients before the advent of the current treatment model. Only on this foundation can we properly interpret the effect of developments in psychiatry that have been so heavily emphasized in other histories of depression.

2

THE MYTH OF THE OLD-TIME DOCTOR

Many people hold to common myths that doctors today have substantially lost their humanistic qualities and that prescribing psychoactive medications is a new approach to treating emotional disorders. In this chapter, we debunk these myths because they distract science and society from confronting more important problems in treating emotional disorders.

There are two reasons to paint an accurate picture of primary-care doctors in the period before researchers developed the current model of depression treatment. First, some critics of the current treatment model suggest that doctors from a bygone era were more likely to treat emotional symptoms with time, empathy, and understanding rather than a reflexive reach for drugs. In this chapter, we demonstrate that data from this earlier time collected specifically to document these factors do not support such a contention. Second, some of the supporters of the current treatment model portray the treatment of emotional symptoms with psychoactive medications as a revolutionary approach. In this chapter, we demonstrate that drug therapy for emotional distress is long-standing.

The Country Doctor

The painting, "The Doctor" (Fig. 2–1) captures one of the most enduring images of the venerated family physician. Henry Tate, a wealthy British art collector,

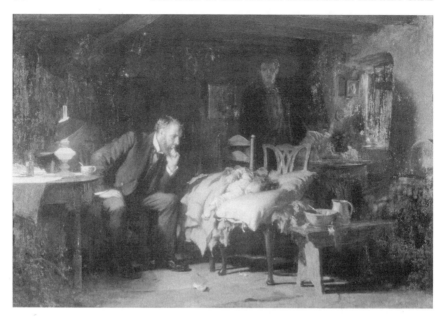

FIGURE 2–1. "The Doctor" by Sir Luke Fildes (1844–1927). Tate Gallery, London/Art Resource, New York.

commissioned Sir Luke Fildes to create the work in 1891. Fildes was inspired by a personal tragedy when he created the image. Although Fildes's son died on Christmas morning in 1877, he was moved by the care and attention that the generalist physician had provided his son and the rest of his family. "The Doctor" portrays a gentle physician waiting dutifully at a girl's bedside in the home of a working-class family. The parents are near a window, which is slightly illuminated by the morning sun. Fildes related that, unlike his son, the young woman in the picture survived, at least into the morning (Wilson 1995). For many patients, this painting conveys the essence of a caring, compassionate doctor: one willing to be with them at home during their most troubled times.

Reproductions of this painting grace the waiting rooms of thousands of primary-care physicians' offices in the United States and the United Kingdom. A U.S. postage stamp even replicated the painting to commemorate the 100th anniversary of the American Medical Association in 1947. Assessing the influence of this image over the past half-century, Gifford (1973) wrote: "Not only did 'The Doctor' serve the patients, it served the physicians too. The painting became an icon of the devoted physician."

"The Doctor" is a romanticized and idealized icon, however. People refer to this medical champion when they nostalgically long for the "old-time country doctor." While many find inspiration in the painting, the sentiment, and the ideal, the truth is that this hero is mythical. Filde's poignant painting, "Applicants for Admission to the Casual Ward" (Fig. 2–2) represents the darker side of this

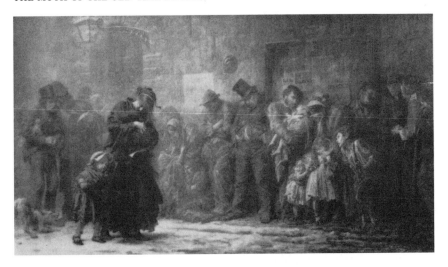

FIGURE 2–2. "Applicants for Admission to the Casual Ward" by Sir Luke Fildes (1844–1927). From L.V. Fildes, *Luke Fildes, R.A.: A Victorian Painter*, Michael Joseph Ltd., 1968.

image, portraying the experience of medical care for most people in the nineteenth century more accurately.

Wilbanks (1972) suggested that nineteenth-century Western art and literature often "glorified a man in his vocation such as the physician, depicting him as a composite of all the qualities possible in a number of people at the peak of perfection." Indeed, after painting "The Doctor," Fildes explained: "I leaned freely on my friends who may have had a feature resembling my ideal . . . and thus compiled from five or six persons 'the Doctor' in the picture as you have him. Many are the letters I have received asking for the name of 'the Doctor'." "The Doctor" never existed. According to Gifford, when Fildes created his painting, patients unrealistically venerated physicians to an unrealistic level as a way of dealing with medicine's ineffectiveness.

Ironically, the public still yearns for this iconic doctor, even though scientists, public health specialists, and physicians have developed increasingly effective remedies against the major causes of mortality. Hoffman (1972) believed the people facing illness amidst the impersonal technology of medicine in the twentieth century often need a scapegoat, and the physician is a logical target:

With old-fashioned traces of the tragic hero buried beneath the modern wave of nonheroes, the doctor in American fiction often aims too high and thus falls further than "the rest of us." But his failure is not only from within; it is from without. His life miscarries as much from society's impossible expectations as from his inability to fulfill society's and his own hopes for his destiny.

These expectations that cannot possibly be achieved emanate from within the profession, as well as without. Educators still promote a mythical "triple-threat" academician as the penultimate ideal of every physician's medical career. A "triple threat" is a physician who achieves and maintains simultaneous excellence in clinical care, trainee education, and medical research throughout his or her entire career. In addition, primary-care physicians are expected to be clinically adept in everything from domestic violence to chemotherapy to diabetes education to preventive health care, pharmacotherapy, clinical research, and on and on. For their part, primary-care physicians and their leadership readily accept this ideal as the reason they chose medicine.

Part of the mystique of this "old family doctor" is how he understands the human condition, his innate listening skills, and his natural ability to provide counseling for a broad range of emotional stresses. Equally essential to this mystique is the doctor's willingness to go to patients' homes whenever needed and to stay for as long as necessary. Some who romanticize this image argue that people were better off with old-time doctors. They hold that the old style of relating to patients helps explain why people in the early twentieth century didn't need psychiatrists or psychoactive drugs and didn't have to endure unnecessary diagnostic tests, surgery, repeated office visits, and needless hospital stays. Indeed, these proponents suggest that the loss of "The Doctor" explains why health-care costs have soared and why patients are so dissatisfied and litigious.

To counteract this myth, we need to develop a more accurate picture of what the medical landscape, health-care system, and physicians were like 50 years ago. At least five detailed descriptive studies have contributed to a clear picture of typical general medicine practices in the 1950s and 1960s in the United States and in the United Kingdom. We review these five studies and provide some supporting evidence from smaller, less comprehensive studies. The goal is to provide a snapshot of general practice at mid-century. We will use this picture to mark the beginning of a journey that ends with the current treatment paradigm for depression in primary care.

Primary-Care Doctors at Mid-Century in the United States

In 1953, Peterson and his colleagues (1956) completed perhaps the most extensive study of day-to-day primary-care practice in the United States. They summarized the study, conducted in North Carolina, as "an attempt to obtain information and understanding about the problems of the general practitioner in the hope that his educational, training, and organizational needs would become clearer." The average number of patient visits to individual physicians per week was 170, or approximately 30 patients a day. These numbers are slightly less than those reported in the United Kingdom at that time, and they are well below the heroic numbers of 50 to 60 patients a day that are often quoted by medical patriarchs. The number of patient visits per week varied among physicians: A small minority of physicians saw 50 patients a day, while the majority saw as many as is typical of a primary-care doctor's practice today—20 to 30 patients.

On average, doctors in the 1950s worked 9.3 hours per day, or about 51 hours a week, including work at an outpatient clinic on Saturday. These 51 hours did not include after-hours calls, however. Using the data from this study, we can estimate that the typical patient visit would have lasted about 15 minutes. The authors suggested that "although these doctors work long, hard hours, [the actual findings regarding the number of hours worked] contrast somewhat with the picture drawn by earlier writers of fact and fiction."

The investigators rated one-third of the physician's offices as unacceptable for patient care. Most of these facilities were superficially remodeled houses (where the doctors and their families lived), with few doctors working in offices specifically built for primary care. The doctor's examination room was typically a side room of the house, and the front parlor served as the waiting room. Laboratory facilities included a microscope, an X-ray machine for chest and extremity radiographs, and an electrocardiograph. Not all practices had this equipment, and facilities for collecting, storing, and analyzing blood samples were unusual. Only 36% of the practices scheduled patient appointments; instead, most relied on the waiting room to regulate patient volume. Most practices employed only one ancillary worker, usually a registered nurse working as a clerk rather than as a health-care provider.

The investigators noted considerable variation in the quality of clinical care that these doctors provided, rating 44% of the physicians as providing poor care, and they documented ineffective history taking and inadequate physical examinations. The investigators summarized the quality of care as follows:

At its very best the practice of medicine resembled that carried out in the medical school. At one extreme, the physician obtained thorough histories and performed careful, competent physical examinations of each patient. The laboratory which was usually manned by a trained professional was used skillfully as an adjunct to practice. Other physician's performances were antipodal. These physicians practiced from their desk chairs. Histories were almost nonexistent and the few questions asked were often irrelevant. Patients were seldom undressed or laid down for an examination.

In particular, primary-care doctors in the 1950s did not pay much attention to examining the heart, which is now regarded as the pinnacle of clinical acumen. Peterson and colleagues reported that only 5% of the physicians displayed "a good complete examination of the heart. The finer points in the technique of auscultation of the heart which may add immeasurably to the amount of information gained in this fashion were not observed during the course of this study." In addition, the researchers documented multiple other deficiencies in the doctors' physical examinations.

The quality of care did not correlate with the size of the practice or with the physician's time pressures (that is, busier physicians were not necessarily low-quality physicians). Also, there was no correlation between quality of care and the physician's frequency of participation in postgraduate education, membership on hospital staff, affiliations with professional organizations, or journal subscriptions. The researchers did report a weak association between the quality of care and the physician's age and performance in medical school, however. The investigators opined that the physicians' personality characteristics had as much to do with the quality of care as traditional sources of medical education did.

Primary-Care Doctors at Mid-Century in the United Kingdom

In the early 1950s, scientists completed several field surveys to assess the state of general practice in England. Joseph S. Collings, a research fellow at the Harvard School of Public Health, conducted the first study. A native Australian, he ultimately pursued a career in general practice in Melbourne (Collings 1950). Collings spent a year in the United Kingdom visiting 104 physicians in 55 separate practices, 30 of which were solo practices. Some of these practices he classified as "industrial," while others were "rural."

Industrial practices were typically located in an inner city area and provided care for a mostly poor, laboring class. These practices are called "surgeries" in the United Kingdom and are equivalent to a general practitioner's ambulatory-care clinic in the United States. Collings (1950) summed up the physical sites of the industrial practices' surgeries as follows:

The adaptation of a shop or a house to a doctor's surgery is usually very elementary. As a rule two adjacent rooms serve as waiting and consulting [examination] rooms, and where dispensing is undertaken, a third room may be set aside for the purpose. That is the basic plan, and there is very little variation from it. . . . Few skilled craftsmen, be they plumbers, butchers, or motor mechanics would be prepared to work under conditions or with equipment as bad (comparably) as that tolerated by many doctors working in industrial practices.

His summation of the quality of care was equally critical:

Under the prevailing conditions of industrial practice, anything approaching a general or complete examination is out of the question; "examinations" are usually confined to the offending organ and even then are cursory. . . . Treatment is even more restricted than diagnosis. Most of it is symptomatic, and nearly all of it is medicinal: for there is neither time nor opportunity for physical therapy or psychotherapy. . . . Medical records are either non-existent or so superficial as to be valueless. The overall state of general practice in England is bad and still deteriorating. Some working conditions are bad enough to require condemnation in the public interest. Inner city practice is at the best unsatisfactory and at the worst a source of public danger.

Industrial practices, located in the shadow of the university-based medical centers, had the worst facilities and lowest quality of care, a finding that contradicted the prevailing notion that urban general practitioners benefited from the facilities of the nearby medical centers. Policy makers at that time believed that general practitioners collaborated closely with the local academic physicians and that city-based doctors benefited from better access to continuing medical education. Collings and others have reported that not only was there poor collaboration between academic medical centers and local general practitioners but the relationship between them was often adversarial.

Collings presented the typical practitioner as beleaguered, demoralized, unappreciated, and looking for a way out, for which he primarily blamed general-practice leadership. He also blamed the leadership and rank and file of other specialty societies, as well as the policy makers who had been entrusted with the responsibility of providing a strong general practice foundation for medical care. The findings from Collings's study were controversial and hotly debated: "There is no doubt that this report both provoked an immediate angry response from the profession and stimulated research" (Morrell 1998). Charles Webster (1988), the official historian of the National Health Service, described Collings's report as "the single most effective factor in mobilizing opinion in favor of constructive change."

In another study, the British Medical Association (BMA) commissioned and funded a field survey of general practice by a General Practice Review Committee led by S. J. Hadfield, a member of the BMA's governing board, in 1951 (Report of the General Practice Review Committee 1953). While Hadfield's findings were more positive than those of Collings, they nonetheless raised many concerns about the state of general practice.

The typical general practice physician in the Review Committee's sample was responsible for 1500 to 2500 patients. A typical morning clinic for these physicians started at 9 a.m., and in the next 90 minutes they saw up to 25 patients: "[The physician] may spend 15 minutes on one patient and then quite appropriately deal with the needs of 5–6 others during the next 15 minutes." The study also found that these practitioners conducted 15 to 30 home visits per day, usually seeing about five patients per hour in homes spread out over a 15- to 20-mile radius. "It is rare that a visit to the house lasts for more than 10 minutes and many need not be so long. There is nowadays little of the old custom of turning the doctor's visit into a social occasion" (Report of the General Practice Review Committee 1953).

The BMA study confirmed that few doctors practiced in buildings purposefully built for medical care: 24% of the physicians had "fairly adequate premises, which, however, lacked some essential such as a wash basin," and 10% had unsuitable and inadequate premises, half of which lacked even an examination couch. The committee judged that 69% of the general practitioners examined patients when it was necessary, 24% took chances and failed to make the necessary examinations, and 7% were "in the danger zone" of never examining patients.

The researchers stated that 75% of the physicians paid a "reasonable amount of attention to record keeping." Most practices did not employ a secretary or nurse, most did not schedule appointments, and the most common ancillary staff was the doctor's wife; many felt professionally isolated. The report concluded that "about half of the general practitioners in the National Health System are reasonably happy and contented in their work and a similar proportion may be described as 'good' doctors."

Although this study's findings were more positive than those in Collings's report, Stephen Taylor (1954), who also completed a survey of general practice physicians in the United Kingdom, pointed out that if 25% of general practitioners were delivering substandard care, "5,000 doctors [were] looking after some 10 million patients. Taking into account the 5% of physicians who were clearly dangerous, "1,000 doctors [were] in charge of some 2 million patients." The United Kingdom viewed the finding that one in four doctors was inadequate as unacceptable. General practice clearly was in need of fundamental reform. On multiple fronts, the leadership of general practice in the United Kingdom set out to stimulate improvement and influence new policy developments. We discuss these changes in Chapter 6.

In Taylor's (1954) survey of general practice in the United Kingdom, conducted in 1953, he aimed to identify and disseminate what we now call "best practices." Taylor's study differed substantially from those of Collings and Hadfield because he sought to "find and describe in detail the best in general practice [to] learn something of value about the organization and conduct of practices. . . . The object was to find examples of successful achievement, particularly examples which could be applied generally." Taylor selected the practices that Hadfield's committee had defined as excellent, and he purposefully selected a sample of 30 of the better-run general practices in England and Wales to conduct his study. He published his findings as a book, *Good General Practice*, a textbook on how to organize and operate an efficient general practice of high quality.

Taylor collected data from 94 physicians in 30 different practices during 1951 and 1952. While the practice sizes averaged 2500 patients per physician, the number of patient visits a day per physician ranged between 27 and 87, with a mean of about 50. Time spent with patients fell into four categories. Doctors handled "quickies," such as medication refills and filling out illness certificates, at a rate of 20 an hour (3 minutes per patient). They also completed follow-up visits and short new cases at a rate of 6 to 12 an hour (5–10 minutes each). Intermediate cases required 15 to 25 minutes each. Patients requiring more than this amount of time required multiple visits or a home visit to not slow down the pace of the clinic. For record keeping, Taylor recommended that a visit "should seldom result in more than five lines" in the medical record. He found that 10% of doctors never made medical record entries for patient visits, and 90% never made medical record notes for home visits.

Although Taylor made no contention that he had assembled a random sample, he did generalize the results when discussing the quality of care in the United Kingdom. He reported that "about one quarter of general practitioners are very good indeed. About one half are good, sound and reliable and one would not hesitate to call them in for one's family. About one-quarter are unsatisfactory with poor equipment and no records." Although Taylor criticized Collings for overgeneralizing from data collected in a biased sample, he could have applied this same criticism to himself. Reacting to Collings's condemnation of many general practitioners' inadequate facilities, Taylor explained as follows:

It is part of the pride of many English doctors, scientists, lawyers, and others that they are oblivious of all but the essentials of their environment. They remember the tradition of string, sealing wax, and plasticine of most of our great English laboratories of physics and physiology. They would suggest that it is quality of mind rather than the trimmings which matters. They view the external manifestations of efficiency as meretricious etceteras, in all probability designed to hide an intellectual vacuum.

Taylor wrote this rejoinder to Collings's contention that most general practitioners had inadequate diagnostic equipment:

Here is a failure to understand an underlying principle of English clinical teaching. Occasionally a microscope is useful to the GP; it is simple to use, and even the occasional user will seldom make mistakes. But most pathological and special tests, including electrocardiography, are only of value in the hands of those who are constantly using them. There are so many traps for the inexperienced person that his results are unreliable. Such results may be positively misleading, by producing a false sense of security.

These quotations demonstrate how easy it is to mislead by stereotypes and fall back on platitudes about the art of medicine in a bygone age. Taylor's failure to adhere to rules of scientific evidence is of concern to us because his goal was to prove that "the picture is far less black than [Collings] painted it" (Taylor 1954). From our perspective in the twenty-first century, all of these reports of general medical care in the 1950s would be viewed as bleak.

As another example of how attitudes change, consider Taylor's genuine attempt to compliment women physicians:

An unusual feature of the practice of the good woman GP is sometimes the large amount of minor surgery done. Such doctors get great pleasure out of removing sebaceous cysts and opening whitlows and abscesses; they do it extremely efficiently; with the neatness, aplomb, and expertise which might otherwise go into dress-making and embroidery.

In another study conducted in several general practices in the United Kingdom, Eimerl and Pearson (1966) observed the amount of time that general practitioners allocated to direct patient care. A typical practitioner in their sample worked a five-and-one-half-day workweek, for a total of 42 hours. On average, he saw 273 patients per week, including both home and office visits, with home visits lasting 15 to 18 minutes, and office visits lasting 5 to 7 minutes. However, the authors noted that the amount of time spent with patients depended on the individual physician's daily workload:

That the pattern of practice should be so rigid is of great interest and significance. Individual practitioners spent much the same time whether seeing 20 patients or 40. Some spent on average 2 minutes per patient in the consulting room in order to make all the consultations within the self-imposed timetable.

Studies of rural physicians in the United Kingdom painted a similar picture of primary-care practice in the 1960s. Bebbington (1969) reviewed 508 consecutive patients seen in a rural practice in North Wales. Each doctor cared for about 2200 patients, and the 508 patients studied represented one month's worth of patients. The investigators estimated that physicians spent about 7 minutes with each patient on average. Bebbington reported a conflict between volume of patients and limited time for preventive health care. With doctors attending to so many patients, Bebbington concluded that

It is clear that there is much serious undiagnosed illness in the community and it can be argued that a general practitioner should be more active in searching for his undiagnosed anemic patients, chronic bronchitics, depressives, and urinary infections than for his one case of cervical cancer every three years.

When people may reminisce about the genteel and humane picture of the general practitioner in the mid-twentieth century, it is important to balance the picture with the criticisms of that time. Critics often reprimanded physicians for their ineffectiveness, as well as their paternalism and complacency. It is impossible to argue that physicians had both greater volume and more time with patients, and there is little evidence that total number of work hours have changed significantly over the past half-century. Data do not support contentions that early to mid-twentieth-century physicians possessed excellent physical examination skills. The truth about the state of general practice in the United Kingdom at mid-century probably lies somewhere between the bleak picture reported by Collings and the sometimes gratuitous picture offered by Taylor and Hadfield. This middle ground is also where Peterson placed the overall quality of care of general practice in the United States.

Satisfaction with Primary-Care Doctors at Mid-Century

What did the general practitioners and their patients think about the problems and prospects of general practice at mid-century? In a survey conducted in the United Kingdom in 1963, Ann Cartwright and her colleagues at the Institute of Community Studies (Cartwright and Marshall 1965; Cartwright 1967) addressed this question. The researchers sought to "describe the care given by the general practitioner service and to discover the attitudes of both patients and doctors to this care."

Cartwright reported that 58% of practitioners estimated that they personally cared for more than 2500 patients. The average number of visits per patient per year was about 4.5. Half of the doctors worked in a solo practice or with just one other partner, and 95% of the physicians were men. Most patients passively chose their doctors either because the physician had taken over their former physician's practice or because the physician was closest in proximity to their home or workplace. About half of the patients typically walked to the doctor's office, and 80% traveled their doctor's office in 15 minutes or less. One-third of the patients had been with their current doctor for less than five years, and one-third of all patients had not seen their physician in the prior 12 months. Only one in 10 practices used an appointment system. In practices with an appointment system, 49% of patients reported that they waited 10 minutes or less to see the doctor; in practices without an appointment system, this proportion was only 18%. However, using an appointment system did not alter the average number of patient visits per year.

About one-half of the physicians reported having a professional affiliation with a local hospital. A large percentage of physicians reported that they never or rarely performed such minor surgical procedures as excising cysts (71%), draining abscesses (48%), stitching lacerations (40%), or performing vaginal speculum examinations (40%). Doctors typically sent patients needing these procedures to the hospital or to a consultant; 60% of patients reported they would go straight to the hospital if they suffered a cut on their leg that needed stitching. Cartwright also reported that general practitioners were not very involved in promoting preventive health measures; they reported that they did not have the staff to participate more actively, even though they recognized that preventive health care was important.

"Unnecessary" consultations were the most frequently reason cited for frustration among general practitioners. Over 50% of physicians estimated that over 25% of patient visits were for trivial reasons; 26% of these physicians reported that over 50% of patient visits were inappropriate. Doctors with the highest estimate of trivial visits also were the most dissatisfied with their vocation, performed the fewest office procedures, attended the fewest educational courses, and reported the lowest self-respect.

About 20% of all visits took place in the patient's home, with the rest occurring in the doctor's office. During the visits, doctors prescribed medication (in 71% of the visits), provided a certificate of health or illness (14%), referred the patient (10%), and gave advice or reassurance (41%). Most patients rated their care as satisfactory and agreed that the services delivered exceeded their expectations. The authors suggested that patient expectations may have been too low or that perhaps patients had been reluctant to criticize their doctors.

Cartwright identified four important characteristics that define a "personal doctor." First, patients felt their doctors would know them by name if they were to meet on the street. Second, the patients would enjoy a friendly, rather than businesslike, relationship with their doctors. Third, the patients would discuss a personal problem with their doctor even if it were not strictly medical. Fourth, the patients felt their doctors would explain health concerns to them fully. While 88% of patients reported that their physicians met one of these criteria, only 11% felt that they met all four criteria. According to Cartwright, there was a passive and uncritical atmosphere among patients and doctors; she argued that this environment might lead to stagnation and stifle quality improvement.

Prescribing Practices of the Old-Time Doctor

These and other observational studies from this period reported that 70% to 95% of patient visits resulted in a drug prescription. In a 1950 study by Brotherston and Chave, among patients visiting a physician at least once during the year, the prescription rate was nearly five prescriptions per patient (Brotherstone and Chave 1956). During only 5% of patients' visits did doctors not prescribe a medication.

What were the physicians prescribing at the turn of the century? In a 1952 study, Dunlop and colleagues described all medicines prescribed from representative areas throughout the United Kingdom. Doctors wrote about 20% of prescriptions for proprietary preparations and the remainder for nonproprietary medications. While many medications could be purchased without a prescription, many patients sought out the doctor's advice and preferred to have a written prescription.

Doctors prescribed sedative-hypnotics more frequently than any other drugs, accounting for 15% of all prescriptions. The most common of these medications were barbiturates (9.4%) and bromides (5.8%), but doctors typically prescribed the bromides in doses too low to be effective. The authors noted that doctors should have avoided bromides because of their side effects and, instead, should have chosen more effective preparations (for example, chloral hydrate or phenobarbitone). Sedative-hypnotics, antacid-type preparations (9%), and tonics (8%) accounted for one-third of all prescriptions. The researchers described tonics as "elegant and complex recipes which are still manifestly popular, although they must generally be classified as placebos."

Antipyretics, cough mixtures, and vitamins accounted for another 20% of prescriptions. In comparison, bronchodilators comprised 4% of prescriptions, and cardiac glycosides and nitrate preparations each accounted for less than 2% of prescriptions. Although the medicines were new to the therapeutic armamentarium in 1949, doctors infrequently prescribed penicillin (4%) and sulfonamides (3%). In addition, they prescribed antibiotics most often as ointments rather than as oral preparations. The authors lamented most doctors' poor pharmacological training, complaining that "many young graduates go into practice with a very inadequate knowledge of applied pharmacology, and tend to rely more and more on the ingenious (sometime very good, but sometimes very misleading) advertisements of the drug firms which cover his breakfast table."

To provide a more complete picture of the therapies that general practitioners employed, Scott et al. (1960) completed a detailed study of the practice patterns of a small group of physicians in 1956–1957. The prescribing rate per patient was 2.5 prescriptions per year. The doctor referred the patient to a nurse in 14% of the visits and to a social worker in 3%. The physician wrote a new prescription during 38% of the visits, but 60% of the visits involved either a new prescription, the continuation of a medication, or a suggestion to obtain a medication. Many of the visits included medical advice or instruction (28%), explanations about health or illness (22%), and joint discussions (18%), though to a far lesser degree, therapeutic listening (3%). The authors noted the substantial volume of personal and social problems that general practitioners addressed and concluded:

Though science has provided the modern family doctor with many more precise and specific cures in the form of powerful drugs which were denied to his predecessors, there is no evidence that proportionately less of his total therapeutic endeavor is concerned with the less tangible problems of fear, pain, personal insecurity, and social maladjustment.

In these audits of primary-care practice at mid-century, it is easy to find similarities and parallels with practice at the beginning of the twentieth century. We stress that there is little hard evidence to indicate the existence of the kind of doctor portrayed in Fildes's painting. Most important, there is little evidence that a loss in physician empathy, clinical skills, counseling abilities, or time explains our current limitations in caring for people with emotional disorders.

Summary

Primary-care practice during the mid-twentieth century would have failed any standard of care that we would find acceptable today. Although most people would agree with this sensibility, some still suggest that the mid-century primary-care doctor's interpersonal attributes would be more desirable than those of today's doctors.

Referring to one of our core arguments: these data show that there has been little change in primary-care doctors' basic approach to patients with emotional symptoms over the past half-century. In later chapters, we trace important changes in the primary-care setting itself, as well as in the diagnosis and treatment of depression. In the following chapter, we build the case for another core argument—namely, that there has been little change in the help-seeking behavior of patients with emotional disorders.

3

THE MYTH OF THE OLD-TIME PATIENT

When public health experts address the limitations of the current model for treating depression in primary care, they sometimes contend that people living 50 years ago had more intestinal fortitude and were less likely to seek medical solutions for their emotional and social problems than people are today. In their view, community resources both prevented and treated emotional symptoms in a manner that rendered these symptoms less disabling. They also contend that these old-time patients were less likely to seek drugs and that patients today are too ready to seek care from physicians for the most minor complaints, including minor emotional symptoms. The goal of this chapter is to counter these myths by describing how often people suffered from emotional disorders at mid-century, how often they sought care, and what types of care they expected to receive from their doctors.

The Stress of War on Civilians

Christopher Wren (1632–1723), an astronomer, mathematician, and architect, designed St. Paul's Cathedral in London. The cathedral's huge, classical dome rises 365 feet above the ground. In a famous photograph taken on December 29, 1940, this dome was the lone structure rising above a sea of flames and smoke. On that night, more than 50 firebombs fell on or near the cathedral. Although a small band of volunteers saved the cathedral from severe damage, bombs destroyed a large part of London that night. In many of the major cities in Eastern England, one can find older stone buildings and monuments that still bear the scars of World War II. Besides air raids, Britain's citizens endured the death and injury of countless family and friends, long hours of work devoted to the war effort, food rationing, fuel rationing, and the imminent threat of invasion. Many people sent their children to North America to keep them safe and redirected their careers to devote their energies to their country's fight for survival.

One such man, Aubrey Lewis, was a psychiatrist from Australia who had trained in the United States, England, and Germany and worked as the clinical director at London's Maudsley Hospital. While at Maudsley, he distinguished himself in research on the history and presenting symptoms of emotional disorders. When the threat of war drew closer to British soil, he remained in London, even as he sent his wife and children to Canada (Shepherd 1977).

Many feared that the cumulative effect of wartime stress would result in more illness, a loss of work productivity, and increased morbidity and mortality in the civilian population. As a result of these concerns, the U.K.'s medical and political leadership conducted a series of population-based surveys to ascertain and monitor the prevalence of sickness in the community. Researchers complemented the community-based surveys with studies conducted in industry, hospitals, and the general practice setting. Lewis organized and participated in several of these early surveys, including a study that examined the impact of psychiatric disorders on work productivity. This attributed social significance to psychological research and treatment: The potential to increase work productivity, including combat productivity, gave credibility to treatments for emotional disorders.

During the war, Lewis (1942) and his colleagues sought to assess the prevalence of neurosis in the civilian population. After the war, Lewis became the director of the Institute of Psychiatry at Maudsley Hospital, which spawned dozens of leaders in education, clinical care, and research in specialty psychiatry. Notably, Lewis also founded the Social Psychiatry Research Unit, which espoused an interdisciplinary approach to psychological illness and designed studies to assess the broader impact of psychiatric morbidity in communities. This unit was one of the first to conduct epidemiological psychiatry and mental health services research, particularly in primary-care settings.

World War II marked a turning point in our understanding of the frequency of relatively minor mental illness. In the United Kingdom, interest in the "minor" forms of depression started after World War I, and by the late 1920s experts described these emotional symptoms as "reactive," "neurotic," and "exogenous" in nature. Consequently, many believed minor depression to be discontinuous from the more severe forms of mental illnesses, such as melancholia and depressive insanity. Lewis first challenged this view in the 1930s, and a debate on the etiology of depression continued into the 1970s (Berrios 1992). Community-based epidemiological studies in the United Kingdom and the United States before this time had focused almost exclusively on the smaller group of patients with the most severe forms of psychiatric illness. Increasingly, scientists began to explore the prevalence of more minor forms of mental illness and the help-seeking behaviors of those affected by them; these studies provide us with information about patients at mid-century.

When interpreting prevalence rates in these studies, it is important to understand how the researchers identified potential subjects. For example, were study subjects volunteers from a psychiatry clinic or a random sample from a defined community? Help-seeking behaviors alter the apparent prevalence of the condition when investigators identify study subjects as only those who seek help from a psychiatrist. Using data from both British and American surveys in the 1950s and 1960s, White et al. (1961) developed a model to describe adults' help-seeking behaviors. Horder (1954) reported similar findings, also using data from the British Survey of Sickness. This research attempted to describe the prevalence of sickness episodes and symptoms based on self-reports from a defined community, rather than from patients seeking care. These researchers stated that in a population of 1000 adults at risk, approximately 750 reported one or more illnesses or injuries a month. Of these, only 250 sought a physician's advice for the illness one or more times a month. Of these 250 patients seeking primary care, doctors admitted nine to a hospital and referred only five to another physician. Among all of these patients, only one received treatment in tertiary care, such as an academic medical center. These scientists concluded that there was an enormous amount of self-care taking place, as well as extensive untreated and inadequately treated illness, including psychiatric illness.

This reservoir of untreated illness in the community, coupled with the reservoir of patients who sought care for symptoms that remained unexplained by their physician, contributed to the frequency of illness over time. In other words, changes in help-seeking behaviors or changes in how physicians label symptoms can alter the apparent rate of illness, even when the true rate has not changed. To extend the analogy of the reservoir: A dam modulates the flow of the river downstream. The operator can open and close the dam gates in a manner that does not necessarily reflect the reservoir's height or the rainfall upstream. In a similar way, as modulators of the rates of mental illness seen in primary care, social forces and health systems have as much control over the gates as scientific forces. To get a true picture of illness rates, then, scientists must go "upstream" and measure symptoms in the community. World War II stimulated the early community-based research in this area.

How Often Did People Get Sick?

During World War II, mental health advocates in the United States and the United Kingdom first became aware of the potential for a huge reservoir of unrecognized psychiatric illness. The United States rejected two million men for military service because of personality or emotional problems revealed through enlistment screening tests (Menninger 1948). These were not men with severe mental illness but, rather, men who occupied a gray zone between mental health and mental illness. As mentioned earlier, the stresses of war also raised concerns about the civilian population's health and productivity. These concerns precipitated several community-based studies that spawned interest in understanding help-seeking behaviors and the epidemiology of emotional problems in primary care.

The Survey of Sickness conducted in the United Kingdom from 1943 to 1952 was an early, community-based survey intended to determine how often people experienced illness, including emotional disorders (Stocks 1949; Logan and Brooke 1957). Scientists designed the survey in order to catalogue patterns of minor illnesses, and they postulated that hardships related to World War II would increase the rates of emotional symptoms. Emotional symptoms at this time were not labeled with the term "depression." Practitioners used terms such as "neurosis" or "psychoneurosis" to describe patients with mild emotional symptoms and to distinguish these symptoms from more severe forms of mental illness, such as psychoses. The use of the word "neurosis" implied that the symptoms originated outside the brain and emanated from nerves. Thus, stress led to an impaired nervous system, rather than a deranged mind. There were no diagnostic criteria for such terms as psychoneurosis, and how physicians used them varied from practice to practice. Such terms were often a diagnosis of exclusion: If a physician could not explain the patient's presenting symptoms, then the symptoms were attributed to psychoneurosis. (The evolution of these terms into our current definition of depression is discussed in Chapter 9.) The Survey of Sickness found that nervous complaints accounted for 247 episodes of illness per 1000 people per month. Ill-defined symptoms and conditions accounted for another 289 episodes. Women were more likely to report nervous complaints, as were those with fewer socioeconomic resources.

Perhaps as surprising as the prevalence of these conditions was the disability associated with them. Nervous complaints accounted for an average of 0.61 days of incapacity per person per month, and ill-defined conditions accounted for another 0.91 days of disability per person per month. Psychoneurosis alone accounted for 361 days of incapacity per 10,000 people per month and 579 doctor visits per 10,000 people per month. The only conditions contributing a greater amount of disability were respiratory diseases and rheumatic conditions (Stocks 1949). These findings presaged those reported by the World Health Organization in 2000, as described in Chapter 1.

In the United States, epidemiologists conducted large-scale studies to describe the frequency and types of illness experienced by representative populations. In particular, these early studies addressed issues related to lost work productivity, the family's role in the genesis and prevention of illness, and the influence of socioeconomic stress as a proximate cause of illness (Collins 1940; Downes 1950; Downes and Simon 1954; Srole et al. 1962). Other studies implemented strategies to identify patients with psychiatric illness among military recruits or other large populations (Weider et al. 1945, 1946; Brodman et al. 1952).

The study in the United States that most closely paralleled the purpose and design of the Survey of Sickness was the Eastern Baltimore Study (Downes 1950; Downes and Simon 1954), in which researchers interviewed nearly 21,000 subjects between 1938 and 1943. Psychoses occurred at a rate of 5.3 cases per 1000 people per year. Psychoneurosis and nervousness occurred at a rate of 15.1 cases per 1000 people per year and resulted in 50 physician visits and 0.8 hospitalizations per 1000 persons per year. About 74% of patients with psychoneurosis saw their physician with these complaints, and doctors referred 12% of such patients to a psychiatrist. Patients with psychoneurosis were more likely to suffer from acute illnesses, including accidents, and were more likely to suffer from chronic medical conditions. Women accounted for 71% of those with psychoneurosis.

In another study, Pasamanick and colleagues (1957) completed a survey of 4000 randomly sampled households, including 12,000 people in Baltimore in 1952, to "determine the prevalence of diagnosed and asymptomatic chronic disease and resulting disability." The study was unique because some of the interviewed patients also completed a clinical examination at Johns Hopkins Hospital. The researchers reported that 9.3% of the community-dwelling, urban population had a mental illness. Psychoneurosis occurred in about 5% of patients, and "psychophysiologic autonomic and visceral disorders (e.g. bodily symptoms such as abdominal pain without an obvious cause) accounted for 3.6%, with the remainder due to psychoses."

The findings from these three studies all suggest that the prevalence rates and burden of emotional disorders at mid-century did not differ significantly from those of today. Patients at mid-century were not immune to, nor were they stoically unimpaired by, emotional symptoms. At the same time, people from this era may not have framed their symptoms as a mental illness, and their physicians may not have labeled them as such. The symptoms themselves, however, were no less frequent than what we see today. We turn now to studies designed specifically to explore help-seeking behaviors for emotional distress.

How Often Did People Seek Help?

Studies at mid-century suggested no systematic differences in how often people sought help for emotional symptoms as compared with today. Several such studies in the United Kingdom and the United States investigated the role of socioeconomic status and the social environment in the genesis of psychoneurosis and people's help-seeking behaviors (Brotherstone and Chave 1956; Srole et al. 1962). By the end of World War II, bombs and fires had destroyed large sections of London, leaving many citizens without homes, jobs, markets, and other fundamental components of a stable social environment. At the same time, many citizens with homes lived in overcrowded conditions that contributed to disease, distress, and crime. Consequently, a major home-building effort started soon after the war, which included developing new suburbs and neighborhoods on the outskirts of London. These planned residential communities made it possible for people to live away from the problems of heavy industry.

Brotherstone and Chave hypothesized that people living in these new communities would be less likely to suffer from neuroses than people living in other communities, but they found no difference (Jeffreys et al. 1960). In summarizing, Brotherstone and Chave stated that among a sample of 1000 community-dwelling adults, one could expect that 670 would report that they were free of emotional symptoms and 250 would report mild neurotic symptoms for which they would not seek formal care. The remaining 80 adults would seek care from their general practitioner for neurotic symptoms. Of these, the practitioner would refer six to psychiatry and send only two to the hospital for psychiatric illness (Brotherstone and Chave 1956). The Midtown Manhattan study in the United States reported a smaller group of symptom-free patients (18%) and larger groups with mild to moderate emotional symptoms (71%) and severe symptoms (10%) (Srole et al. 1962).

In the United States, Gurin et al. (1960), under the direction of the Joint Commission on Mental Health and Illness, conducted a survey of Americans' perceptions about their mental health, as well as their help-seeking behaviors. A representative sample of 2460 adults completed the survey; 35% described themselves as very happy, 54% reported that they were pretty happy, and 11% were not too happy. Respondents also were asked to identify the source of their happiness or unhappiness. The greatest source of happiness was central life relationships. This included marriage, children, and family. Issues within the home, such as marriage, children, family, and income, were the sources of both the greatest happiness and the greatest unhappiness, however. One-quarter of respondents also reported a problem for which they felt professional help would be useful. Only 14% sought help, and of these, 42% sought help from clergy, 29% from their general practitioner, 18% from psychiatrists, and 10% from social agencies. Among those seeking help from clergy or their general practitioner, 65% reported that it had helped, while among those seeking care from psychiatrists, only 46% reported that it had helped.

In the United Kingdom, Wadsworth and colleagues (1971) conducted a large study of self-care and help-seeking behaviors using a random sample of 2153 Londoners in 1963. Slightly more than half of the subjects had seen a general practitioner in the past 11 months, and an additional 25% had seen their doctor in the past year. However, only 20% had sought the advice of their doctor for symptoms they had experienced in the past two weeks, and another 15% sought a nonmedical person's advice. The rest relied on self-care, which typically involved rest and self-medication with symptomatic remedies. Physicians prescribed only 33% of ingested medications. These investigators concluded that, contrary to the popular notion that people contact their physicians for any minor complaint, many people engaged in self-care. In fact, in the investigators' view, an important group of patients needed medical care but did not request it. The findings are even more notable because all participants had access to care through the United Kingdom's National Health Service.

In 1975, a team of general practitioners sought to describe the determinants of medical help-seeking behaviors among a random sample of 516 middle-aged women (Banks et al. 1975). On average, this group of women sought medical care for only about one out of every 37 symptoms they experienced. However, the investigators discovered a large disparity in the likelihood of particular symptoms precipitating a visit to a primary-care physician. For example, there were 456 episodes of a "change in energy" for every one physician visit for this complaint. The ratio for headache was 184:1, backache 52:1, limb pain 49:1, and psychological problems 46:1. People often relied on self-care or informal sources rather than the formal health-care system. Writing in the *Annals of Internal Medicine*, the researchers concluded:

An estimated 70–90% of all self-recognized episodes of sickness are managed exclusively outside the perimeter of the formal health care system. In all cases of sickness, the "popular" and "folk" sectors (self-treatment, family care, self-help groups, religious practitioners, heterodox healers, and so forth) provide a substantial proportion of health care. Once this fact is brought into focus, it becomes evident that the professional health care system neither can nor should be expanded to take over this broader area of management. (Kleinman et al. 1978)

Combining these findings with physicians' perceptions that 25% or more of patients who do visit general practitioners present with trivial complaints, we highlight the substantial discordance in opinion about who needs health care. There has been and remains a large reservoir of symptoms and illness in the community. Thus, even minor changes in help-seeking behaviors among the patients constituting this large reservoir have huge implications for the types of illnesses and complaints seen in the formal health system. These changes can readily occur with no change in the background prevalence of illness. In addition, minor changes in how physicians label the large reservoir of nonspecific symptoms have important implications for the apparent prevalence of disease and may precipitate changes in patients' help-seeking behaviors.

How Frequent Were Emotional Disorders in Primary Care at Mid-Century?

Turning from community-based surveys to those conducted among attendees in general medicine clinics, researchers next documented the reasons people sought medical care and estimated how this translated into the typical general practitioner's workload (Backett et al. 1954; Brotherstone and Chave 1956). In the United States, data from the Health Insurance Plan of Greater New York (1948–1951) showed that the most common reasons for physician visits were respiratory conditions, trauma, psychoneurosis, skin disorders, hypertension, and peptic ulcers (Baehr 1950; Densen et al. 1960; Huntley 1963). Allen and Kaufman (1948), in one of the first studies of the prevalence of psychiatric disorders in a general medicine practice, analyzed 1000 patients for emotional complaints and disorders. For 59.4% of these patients, clinicians adjudged the patient's complaints as explained solely by a physical disorder. In 27.2%, the complaints originated solely from a neuropsychiatric disorder, and the remaining 13.4% came from a combination of physical and psychiatric conditions. Other studies from this time period placed the prevalence of emotional disorders in primary-care clinics as high as 80% (Pemberton 1949; Watts and Watts 1952; Fry 1957; Kaufman and Bernstein 1957).

The prevalence of emotional distress in primary care was so high that some investigators began to hypothesize that emotional distress, rather than physical symptoms, was the trigger for seeking medical care. Stoeckle and colleagues (1964) explored the influence of psychiatric distress on the help-seeking behaviors of patients attending a general medicine outpatient clinic at Harvard Medical School in 1958. A general practitioner and a sociologist independently assessed the patients. According to the sociologist, 88% of women and 79% of men were experiencing psychological distress, which was defined by a patient reporting nervousness, a current life stressor, or the patient's responses. Similarly, the physician reported that 87% of the patients had psychological distress, which in 60% of the cases included a depressive reaction. Among other findings, the clinicians concluded that patients' psychological and medical states influenced their decisions to seek care. They suggested that this may have explained why such a large percentage of patients attending primary-care clinics reported emotional distress.

The substantial variation in the reported prevalence rates of emotional disorders in these early studies was a source of much discussion. Kessel and Shepherd (1962) and Shepard et al. (1966) reviewed more than 20 studies conducted between 1949 and 1963 that reported psychiatric morbidity among patients registered in a general practice or consulting a general practitioner. These investigators found widely disparate results, with prevalence rates varying between 3.7% and 53.7%. They concluded that this disparity was mainly caused by differences in methodology, including the sampling procedure, diagnostic classification, threshold of severity defining a case, recording procedures, and data analysis. For example, some investigators included only those with "conspicuous psychiatric morbidity," while others included patients with more minor symptoms or those presenting with conditions believed to be primarily psychosomatic (including asthma and peptic ulcer disease). Researchers completed most of these studies in a single clinic and often relied simply on a single clinician's medical records. Thus, the results reflected not only the local population's help-seeking behaviors but also the physician's practice and diagnostic style and the vagaries of his or her medical record notations. Kessel, Shepherd, and other scientists investigating the epidemiology of mental health in general practice began to point out the limitations of these types of studies and to propose more rigorous methodologies (Howard 1959; Lees and Cooper 1963).

When Shepherd and colleagues (1964) conducted a survey in London that was specifically designed to determine the frequency of emotional disorders in a general practice setting, they found considerable variations in diagnostic thresholds. Although physicians had received instructions in the study's purpose and conduct, they displayed no standardized method of elucidating or recording presenting signs and symptoms and showed no evidence of a set of standardized criteria to define who had an emotional disorder. In other words, diagnosis had a large, subjective component. The authors reported:

There was a widespread tendency to exclude the possibility of serious organic disease before considering the positive indications of a psychiatric diagnosis. While this may be a necessary stage in the transaction between a doctor and patient, with some of the survey doctors it was carried to an extreme. Even when the likelihood of major disease had been eliminated they continued to seek an organic cause for symptoms, and only when patients failed to respond to medication and continued to complain did they begin to think in psychological terms. Thus, a psychiatric diagnosis was often reached only after a period of time and the elimination of other possibilities.

The doctors often failed to recognize or inquire about social stressors and were unaware of the patients' social conditions, even after multiple visits. Even when they recognized these stressors, the physicians only intervened for problems that they thought they could fix. This finding was true for patients presenting psychiatric and psychosomatic disorders as well. Physicians were more likely to make a particular diagnosis when they felt that could offer an effective treatment. The authors also found differences in physicians' ability to communicate with patients from lower social strata. These patients were more suspicious of psychiatry. The authors reported that, among the 2245 patients who completed a standardized questionnaire, 7% of men and 13% of women reported symptoms of depression. Doctors identified less than half of these patients as psychiatric cases. Psychiatric illness was the fourth leading cause of patient visits, behind respiratory conditions, trauma, and dermatologic conditions.

The prevalence of psychiatric morbidity varied substantially across the 50 clinical practices studied, even when using standardized criteria. Shepherd and his colleagues attributed these large differences in the reported prevalence of psychiatric disorders to a combination of random fluctuations, recording errors, true differences in prevalence across practices, and differences in diagnostic practices.

Differing rates of diagnosis for neurosis and psychosomatic conditions largely explained the differences in diagnostic patterns, however.

Importantly, these studies provide evidence that the level of psychiatric morbidity in primary care prior to the advent of the current depression treatment model did not differ significantly from its current level. In the words of a clinician and researcher who has worked in the trenches of primary care throughout the past half century: "Contrary to some expectations, there has been no increase in the prevalence of psychiatric disorders in my practice for over 30 years—it has remained steady at around 10% of all consultations in any and every year" (Fry 1982).

These findings also suggest that people at mid-century were no more or less likely to experience depression and seek help for it than are people today. However, we might wonder why the prevalence of these disorders has not substantially *decreased*. One might posit that emotional disorders should be much less common today, given the massive improvements in public health over the past century. While the incidence of most infectious diseases has fallen markedly with improved standards of nutrition, hygiene, and medical treatment, there is no evidence that the general improvements in living conditions in modern, industrial society have brought about any corresponding decrease in neurotic illness (Kedward and Cooper 1966). The same studies discussed above also documented poor-quality care. We next describe the treatments that patients could expect when they sought care for emotional symptoms, which is important in understanding patients' decisions about when to seek care.

A Void in the Standard of Care at Mid-Century

The general practitioners' explicit role in caring for patients with emotional disorders remained undefined from the end of World War II until at least 1975. In a speech before the New York Academy of Medicine in 1945, Dr. Thomas Rennie (1946), a psychiatrist at Cornell University Medical College, commented:

Until the practitioner's attitude toward psychotherapy can be brought to one of constructive optimism, little can be expected from him as a therapist. . . . If his attitude is primarily disdain and annoyance toward neurotic patients, he should not try to treat them. He need not be seriously concerned about psychiatric diagnostic terms. Diagnoses are at best convenient labels. They add little to the patient's understanding of himself. . . . The diagnosis of psychoneurosis can badly frighten a patient who has heard so much about it in these years of war.

Such comments belie some of the tensions between the unarticulated and ambiguous roles of general practitioners and psychiatrists in treating the large number of patients with emotional disorders presenting to primary-care clinics. Unequivocally, academia's official pronouncement from the 1940s through the 1970s was that the overwhelming majority of these patients should be treated with psychotherapy. One did not have to look far, however, to find derisive comments from psychiatrists themselves about the practicality of psychotherapy. In their book on physical methods of treatment in psychiatry, Sargant and Slater (1954) suggested that psychotherapy was less well studied than the newer, physical methods of treatment. These authors prominently quoted Lord Moran's Presidential address to the Royal College of Physicians in 1945:

The physician of to-day is twice as well equipped in the war with disease as he was when I was a student. And the physician who knows what is wrong with the patient and has an effective remedy in his hands can cut the cackle. He has no need of it.

Even the leadership of British and American psychiatry raised measured concerns about the variability in the wide range of available psychotherapies (Lewis 1953; Appel 1954). For example, Lewis not only raised questions about the efficacy of psychotherapy, but he also criticized the lack of any attempt to identify its active components and to submit it to more rigorous evaluation. In the 1950s and 1960s, psychotherapy became synonymous with psychoanalysis; thus, psychotherapy in general suffered from the negative criticisms and declining confidence expressed toward psychoanalysis. It is hardly surprising that general practitioners were both skeptical and confused about psychotherapy's role in treating emotional disorders in general practice. The ambiguity surrounding which patients with emotional disorders should receive what therapy fostered a conservative and expectant approach by the typical practitioner.

Psychiatry was unsuccessful in demonstrating the practicality of psychotherapy in primary-care settings. Experts failed in the challenge of balancing specific training in psychotherapy with the realities of the primary-care environment. Pragmatic advice often boiled down to fundamentals such as (*a*) listen to the patient to identify the conflict situation, (*b*) gain insight into how this conflict acts on the patient's mind and body, (*c*) convey this insight to the patient, and (*d*) help the patient to readjust and move forward (Bauer 1953). Physicians often confused informal counseling, advice, and reassurance with "psychotherapy" and reported that they naturally always provided such interventions to their patients. There are no data on the effectiveness of these informal physician–patient discussions on the course and outcome of emotional disorders. Michael Balint (1957), a Hungarian refugee who developed his own brand of psychotherapy in England, described these interactions as follows:

No guidance whatsoever is contained in any text-book as to the dosage in which the doctor should prescribe himself, in what form, how frequently, what his curative and his maintenance doses should be, and so on. . . . The usual answer is that experience and common sense will help the doctor to acquire the necessary skill in presenting himself.

"Advice" is usually a well-intentioned shot in the dark, is nearly always futile, and that applies even more strongly to "reassurance."

Balint and his colleagues developed a seminar series to train general practice physicians in simple and pragmatic forms of psychotherapy. Balint decried the inadequate training in psychotherapy and the underuse of the technique, even among psychiatrists. The widespread adoption by general practitioners seemed even more unlikely. Indeed, Balint and his pupils found that training general practitioners in these principles increased their physical and emotional workload, even though doctors found using them professionally rewarding.

Ambivalence regarding the need for active treatment of minor emotional distress, including neurosis and depression, has been an enduring, and at times divisive, attitude in primary care. In the 1950s, opinion leaders described the standard of care for treating neurosis in general practice as symptomatic, supportive, and expectant. Authors tended to stress the self-limited nature of these conditions and the healing passage of time (Brown 1947; Lemere 1957). John Fry, a national opinion leader among British general practitioners, authored a popular textbook, *Common Diseases: Their Nature, Incidence, and Care*, which he first published in 1974 and then updated in multiple, subsequent revisions. We excerpt the treatment recommendation for depression below as a concrete example of expert opinion at this time. This excerpt followed a discussion stressing the importance of a supportive patient-physician relationship and the primacy of counseling and reassurance:

Most patients with depression will recover without serious difficulties and it is well to remember this before deciding to treat all patients with depression with antidepressants. If the depression is not severe and if there are underlying causes that can be defined, discussed, and corrected, then it is reasonable to wait for a little while (2–3 weeks) in order to see whether there is improvement with support and mild sedatives, such as amylobarbitone and hypnotics.

In the textbook's 1979 edition, Fry replaced the phrase "improvement with support and mild sedatives, such as amylobarbitone and hypnotics" with "improvement with support and regular psychotherapy." These 1979 recommendations remained unchanged in the 1983 and 1985 editions.

Most authorities writing on the neurotic patient in primary care recommended rapport and psychotherapy, plus medications, to help treat some of the more troublesome symptoms associated with emotional disorders. For sleep disturbances associated with depression, Watts and Watts (1952) recommended a barbitone solution; for people with more difficult cases of insomnia, they recommended a tonic that combined potassium bromide, chloral hydrate, opium, and aqueous chloroformis, and they identified amphetamine as a potential euphoriant. In 1957, Lemere offered a combination of amphetamine (a stimulant) plus amobarbitol (a sedative) as a potential treatment for depression. He clearly noted, however, that "no drug has been developed that will satisfactorily relieve depression." He identified reserpine and chlorpromazine, both of which had recently become available, as drugs that would aggravate depression. Doctors prescribed these symptomatic medications frequently, and patients expected and requested such remedies when they sought care for emotional symptoms (Dunlop et al. 1952).

There was little or no agreement on diagnostic categories or disease classifications, no suitable control populations, and no standardized outcome measures that might have enabled a systematic investigation of the efficacy of these treatments. In the early 1950s, all of these fundamental requirements for determining which patients should receive which treatments were still awaiting discovery. In his presidential address at the 1952 Annual Meeting of the American Psychopathological Association, Joseph Zubin (1954) remarked:

A great difficulty facing all therapeutic investigations is the question of criteria of improvement. The greatest need of the day is the provision of methods for selecting homogenous groups of patients for evaluation of therapy and for the development of standard control groups which can serve as baselines for the evaluation of new therapies.

How Were Patients Seeking Care Treated at Mid-Century?

Given this cloudy state of affairs regarding the standard of care, how were general practitioners providing for the care of patients with emotional disorders in the 1950s? Shepherd and his colleagues (1966) in their study of 80 general practitioners caring for 15,000 patients, reported that doctors frequently used advice and counseling to treat patients with emotional disorders. The authors found that 28% of patients with diagnosed psychiatric disorders received no treatment at all, and doctors referred only 5% of patients to a psychiatrist. They treated about 33% with a sedative, nearly 20% with a tranquilizer, and 10% with a stimulant, tonic, or placebo. Doctors provided "reassurance," in addition to medications, in about 25% of patients. Fewer than 5% of these general practitioners treated patients with psychotherapy.

In one study (Peterson et al. 1956), primary-care physicians recognized emotional problems and provided competent treatment for only 17% of the patients who warranted it. The investigators reported that doctors failed to recognize emotional problems in 29% of the cases, and for 54% of patients with recognized emotional problems, doctors provided no specific treatment:

Emotional problems constitute an enigma for the practicing physician; many physicians failed to recognize these problems in their practices. Others, while recognizing the problems, were either indifferent to them or appeared to be made uncomfortable by patients with such problems. References to malingering, hypochondriacs, problem patients or getting them out of the office quickly were frequently heard. . . . In actual practice, management of such patients usually involved an extended search for organic disease or repeated prescriptions for a variety of drugs, principally vitamins, iron, antacids, sex hormones, and antispasmodics.

Scott et al. (1960) described the treatment provided for 771 patients whose general practitioners had diagnosed them with "psychoneurosis." In this study, doctors diagnosed 66% of patients based on their history only (i.e., they performed no physical examination). Doctors prescribed medication to 60%, explained the diagnosis to 26%, referred 13% to social services, discussed stress at work with 9%, discussed problems in their personal relationships with 17%, provided therapeutic listening to 29%, and referred 2% to a specialist (with some patients receiving more than one action from their doctor).

In another study, Fink and colleagues (1967) described the treatments prescribed for emotional disorders by 32 family-practice physicians in New York City. Among their 422 patients whom they had diagnosed with psychiatric illnesses, the physicians had prescribed medications to 78% and referred 24% to psychiatry. Nearly 40% of the diagnosed patients reported that they had had no discussion or only a short discussion with their physician about the diagnosis.

Taken together, these four studies show that physicians at mid-century were not regular purveyors of formal or informal psychotherapy. We found no evidence that large numbers of general practitioners attended seminars, such as those designed by Balint, or that educators had altered graduate training to include more instruction in psychotherapy. In short, psychotherapy did not play a significant role in primary-care physicians' treatment of emotional problems at mid-century; instead, symptomatic medications played the major role. Thus, outcomes in primary care for patients with emotional disorders were understandably poor. For example, in Kedward and Cooper's (1966) report of three-year outcomes among 356 patients from 13 general medicine practices in the United Kingdom, only 28% experienced a recovery, and the authors considered 48% unimproved.

To bring the confusion full circle, the authors of a review article on the treatment of mild depression in the *Journal of the American Medical Association* commented that "because of the relative inadequacy of drugs, the main attack on this disease still has to be psychotherapeutic" (Kaufman and Bernstein 1957). The recommendations of this article and dozens of other such pronouncements from academia highlighted the conundrum that emotional problems presented to primary-care physicians and their patients. Multiple authorities in the postwar period espoused psychotherapy for treating emotional problems in primary care (Menninger 1947a; Watts and Watts 1952; Lemere 1957). General-practice physicians, however, had neither the time nor the training to deliver it. As shown in the observational studies discussed in this chapter, researchers found no evidence that primary-care physicians engaged in psychotherapy on any significant scale. Multiple textbooks of medicine, general practice, and psychiatry in general practice, as well as clinical review articles from the 1950s, advocated psychotherapy for patients with emotional disorders. Nevertheless, most of the studies that recorded primary-care physicians' actual practices showed that, at best, patients on both sides of the Atlantic received informal counseling, advice, and reassurance, plus a symptomatic medication for their emotional complaints.

Summary

Three primary findings emerged from these studies with regard to patients and their help-seeking behaviors at mid-century. First, patients, physicians, science, and society disagreed about which human ailments needed formal medical treatment. Many people who seemed to need medical attention did not seek care in the formal health-care system. Instead, many individuals engaged in self-care or sought alternative or complementary care. In addition, numerous providers thought that many people who sought formal health care did not need it. Thus, having access to primary care did not necessarily overcome barriers to seeking help or to treatment. Emotional disorders generated a discord between perceived need, actual need, and help-seeking behaviors.

Second, emotional disorders accounted for a large proportion of disability and were among the most frequent reasons why patients sought care from general practitioners. Mild to moderate mental disorders (as opposed to severe mental disorders) accounted for most disability due to mental illness on a community-wide scale. Third, general-medicine physicians tended to treat psychiatric illness by ruling out biological causes first, and they offered biomedical forms of treatment much more frequently than they did psychosocial interventions. We stress that patients' help-seeking and doctors' treatment patterns were closely linked; it is difficult to separate one from the other.

These fundamental findings continued to resonate for the next half-century through dozens of research studies on patients' help-seeking behaviors and physicians' treatment patterns for emotional disorders. Notably, researchers established each of these findings by the 1950s, even though scientists repeatedly rediscovered, refined, and reinforced them over the subsequent 50 years. The data presented in this chapter addressed the second set of core arguments in our story of reinventing depression. British and American citizens in the 1950s were no less afflicted with emotional symptoms than we are in the early twenty-first century, and they were just as likely to seek care. When they sought care, they had expected drug treatment rather than psychotherapy. Drug therapy with nonspecific psychoactive medications was the most frequently prescribed therapy.

The overall environment and treatment approach of primary care influenced how patients sought care and how doctors provided care for emotional problems. In the next chapter, we piece together a composite picture of primary care in the 1950s to portray the primary-care practice of emotional disorders in context. We also address the question of why people continue to espouse a romantic view of general practice when the data repeatedly refute this ideal.

4

A MORE ACCURATE PICTURE OF PRIMARY
CARE AT MID-CENTURY

This chapter uses the data presented in Chapters 1, 2, and 3 to paint a composite picture of what primary-care practice was like in 1950. When we look too narrowly at the care of emotional disorders, we artificially simplify the complexity of primary care, as well as the challenges that primary-care doctors and patients face when they determine the best approach to treatment. Espousing a romanticized picture of patients and providers at mid-century keeps us from reinventing depression in a useful way because it assumes capacities, talents, and resources that did not exist.

A Day in the Life of a Primary-Care Doctor

Based on studies from the period, we can piece together a reasonably accurate picture of what general practice and general practitioners were like at mid-century. Picture yourself in 1955 as a 45-year-old general practitioner working in a small town, perhaps 25 to 50 miles from the nearest hospital. In all likelihood, you would be practicing alone or in a group of two or three physicians. Whether having been assigned a panel of patients in the National Health Service or operating a fee-for-service practice in the United States, you would care for approximately 2000 patients, each of whom would consult you about four times a year. This would result in about a 50- to 60-hour workweek. You would have extraordinary weeks during which this workload might increase as much as 25%. On an average day, you might see about 20 patients in their homes and 20 patients in your clinic.

Translating this workload to a typical day, you arise at 6 a.m. and begin making half a dozen house calls at 7 a.m. You spend less than 15 minutes in each home and arrive at your clinic at 9 a.m. Your clinic is a wood-framed, two-story house constructed in the late nineteenth century. You pay a mortgage. There is no air-conditioning, private offices, or parking lot. You do not employ a nurse, a medical records clerk, a phlebotomist, or any other health professionals. Your junior partner and his wife live on the second floor of this office, and his wife works as the unpaid receptionist. You and your wife escaped this role only four years ago. There is one telephone that sits near the receptionist's desk in the front parlor. Patients do not make appointments. The practice keeps patient records on small cards filed in alphabetical order, which are stored near the receptionist's desk. Most notations in these medical records consist of the presenting complaint, a diagnosis, and occasionally documentation of the dispensed medication. You do not keep patient notes for home visits, there are no hospital discharge summaries, and it is unusual for consultants to send you records of their assessments.

A converted parlor and an adjoining dining room serve as the waiting area, which is complete with a collection of various wooden chairs and benches. There are two examination rooms, which are furnished with a bookcase, a writing desk, two chairs, and an examination table. The examination table is a low, narrow, wooden table. The practice owns a sphygmomanometer (for measuring blood pressure), a microscope, and a small surgical kit. There is no electrocardiogram, centrifuge, or phlebotomy equipment, and no radiology or laboratory equipment. You complete minor surgical procedures only when the waiting room is not too full. Otherwise, you refer patients requiring surgical procedures to the hospital.

Your partner's wife had begun seating patients in the waiting room at 8 a.m., and there are now about 20 patients already waiting. More will arrive over the course of the morning. Your junior partner started seeing patients one hour ago, while your senior partner attends a home birthing. When all three physicians are in the office, a small study in the rear of the house serves as a third consulting room, but its size precludes any physical examination.

Over the next two and one-half hours, you see 20 patients, spending approximately 5 to 10 minutes with each. You give only four patients more than an organ-specific physical examination, if any, and you make no written medical notes on any patient until lunchtime. You do write a short note of referral for one patient, who you suggest needs to see a cardiologist at the hospital in the next town. Your partner's wife makes lunch at noon. She also brings you the records of the patients you have seen, and you make clinical notes during lunch. After lunch, you see another 10 patients in the early afternoon. One of these patients requires an incision and drainage of an abscess, which you perform without assistance after collecting all the instruments and supplies.

Another patient needs to have a wrist fracture stabilized. He is a widower, and you call your wife to drive him to the hospital. By 2 p.m. you have left the junior partner to finish seeing the remaining patients, and you resume your home visits. You visit another five homes, where you see eight different patients. You arrive back at your home before 6 p.m., having met face-to-face with 44 patients. You spend several hours that evening working on bills to patients, which you send out three or four times per year, and you have a collection rate of about 70%. That night, four telephone calls interrupt your sleep, none of which requires you to leave home, though you add one of the callers to tomorrow's morning house calls. This is a typical day.

Of the 44 patients, you diagnose 20% with upper respiratory symptoms, most of which you consider self-limited, though you prescribe symptomatic treatment. Dermatologic conditions, various digestive complaints, and psychiatric illness each account for 10% to 15% of the visits. You prescribe nearly all of these patients a medication and give half some additional advice, education, or counseling. Your patients are generally happy with your care, but you and your colleagues all harbor a chronic, low-grade sense of deprivation and demoralization. These feelings arise from a perception that your day-to-day routine conflicts with your notion of a high-quality and personally rewarding clinical practice. You have little time for preventive health, formal counseling, continuing medical education, or community activism. Also, both you and your family feel that your time available for family, hobbies, and holidays is inadequate. You feel you are well compensated for your clinical care, but not for your frustration.

Facing the Real Picture of Primary Care at Mid-Century

Around the time of World War II, British general practice was characterized as follows: "The one-minute consultation, the bottle of medicine, and the long queue around the corner out of the surgery door were the daily reality of a service under great strain" (Bosanquet and Salisbury 1998). To "see" 60 to 80 patients in a single day, general practitioners met face-to-face with each patient for less than five minutes. Thus, while the physician's volume of patients may seem impressive, one must be realistic about what was obviously *not* happening during such visits.

Even as late as 1960, physicians experienced frustration because of their inability to do more for their patients. David Morrell (1998), whose career in general practice spanned the second half of the twentieth century, bemoaned the lack of specific therapies:

Pulmonary tuberculosis was still taking young lives, and poliomyelitis was a constant anxiety in the summer months. There was no effective treatment for hypertension, schizophrenia, asthma, or depression, and the management of peptic ulcer was bedrest, alkali, and very often surgery. The management of heart failure depended on digitalis and painful injections of mersalyl, and rheumatic heart disease was still responsible for many being crippled by cardiac failure.

In hospital practice, doctors had become accustomed to using X-rays and laboratory tests to help solve clinical problems. In many areas of the country, particularly in the immediate vicinity of teaching hospitals, these facilities were denied to general practitioners, because the specialists were not convinced that they would use them responsibly, or be capable of interpreting the results. It was not surprising that in the 1950s there were many angry general practitioners, expected to undertake an excessive workload and deprived of adequate resources in order to fulfil a role which had not been properly defined and for which they had not been trained.

Before World War II, physicians had little influence over the course of most diseases. Julian Tudor Hart (1994), another British general practitioner whose career nearly spanned the last half century, suggested:

It is generally agreed by historians that not until the early years of the twentieth century did all medical and surgical intervention put together even begin to save more lives than they destroyed. Substantial net saving of life began only about 1935, with the introduction of sulphonamide antibiotics. [By 1948] medical care was rapidly shifting from dominant illusion sustained by scraps of reality to dominant reality contaminated by residual illusion.

The point of creating an accurate portrayal of general practice at mid-century is not to glorify or to degrade the general practitioners' talent and dedication. Rather, the point is that current leaders, physicians, and patients often wax nostalgic about a golden era of "old-time doctors" that never existed. Although he lamented the decline in the one-on-one relationship between a physician and patient, Ronald Gibson (1981), a leader in British general practice put it this way: "There must be no further harking back to the good old days for time has proved that they were far from good in many respects."

Confronting the Myth of "the Doctor"

Given the data available based on direct observations of clinical practice, why does the image of the old country doctor endure? One simple answer is our dissatisfaction with the current system of care. This dissatisfaction drives a longing for a simpler time that is largely imaginary. When provided with evidence that the old country doctor is mythical, commentators often simply refer to an earlier era when real data were even more elusive. For example, they might argue that perhaps doctors in the 1950s had already lost the art of patient–physician communication, but doctors before World War II still had those extraordinary qualities.

Edward Shorter (1985), a professional historian who submitted himself to part-time medical school training for four years, defended such a view. According to his perspective, the growing conflict between physicians and patients and the perceived increasing dissatisfaction of patients about their physicians' interpersonal skills had three causes. First, physicians in the 1920s and 1930s simply spent more time with their patients, did not rush them, and were more empathetic listeners. Second, physicians were more adept at both recognizing the distress of the vicissitudes of life and using their position of influence to effect a placebo response. Third, patients were less likely to interpret their symptoms as a disease, had greater social support, and were thus less likely to seek care for common symptoms, especially those originating from psychological distress. Considering that Shorter's point of view contradicts our argument, it is useful to submit his supporting evidence for these three claims to closer scrutiny.

Shorter argued that doctors of the 1920s and 1930s devoted quite a bit of time to each patient. The only objective research that Shorter provided to support this claim was an account from the U.S. Public Health Service for the period of 1928–31, which reported that the average number of visits for a typical illness was 3.6. Shorter also noted the substantial proportion of visits conducted in the home and listed a series of quotations and recommendations from medical textbooks of the period. The textbooks suggested that physicians should spend time listening to their patients and included anecdotes from physicians' biographies that detailed the time spent on particular patients by individual physicians. These data fall far short of providing explicit evidence that doctors of the 1920s were better listeners than those in the 1950s or 1990s, or that they spent more time with patients. Shorter allowed:

I don't think the distribution of generosity, charitableness, or general niceness has shifted much in the medical profession over the centuries, just as it has changed very little in most of mankind over that time. I shall not be suggesting that a deterioration of medical character or of morality is responsible for the almost brutal brevity of many consultations today.

Undoubtedly, findings from other studies, such as those by Peterson et al. (1956) and Hadfield (1953) in the 1950s cited in the previous chapter, dispelled any myths about how much time the typical general practitioner spent in an average patient visit soon after World War II. Systematic and objective data from the 1920s about the content and duration of visits are simply not available. However, the public's general view of physicians in the period around 1920 was ambivalent at best. There were severe problems in the distribution of physicians and inadequate access to care for the poor; and there was a nearly complete lack of attention to preventive health, health education, and mental health. Without knowing what proportion of the poor lacked access to medical care before the twentieth century, it is difficult to make sense of attendance figures quoted for these earlier periods. There were also criticisms and concerns about physicians' ability to communicate with patients (Moore 1927). This was a period of patent medicines, competing guilds of practitioners, and a wide variety of alternative medical therapies. Fear of doctors was likely as prevalent as satisfaction with doctors.

For patients with mental illness in particular, it is clear that primary-care physicians in the early part of the twentieth century had no special skills, training, or empathy.

Cuthbert A. H. Watts, a general practitioner in the United Kingdom who trained in the 1930s and had a long career as a general practitioner, conveyed this view. During World War II, Dr. Watts completed additional training in psychiatry and completed some of the early textbooks on the care of psychiatric illness in primary care (Watts and Watts 1952; Watts and Stengel 1966). He describes the care of psychiatric patients in the 1930s and 1940s:

Few of us who qualified in the middle thirties found ourselves equipped with any knowledge of psychiatry. In the years after graduation when I was a houseman, few psychiatric cases came my way in the highly selected hospital population and I was kept blissfully unaware of any need for experience in this field. Medicine in those hospital days was almost completely an affair of organic disease, and any psychiatric casualty was viewed as the usurper of a useful hospital bed—something to be removed with almost unseemly haste. (Watts and Watts 1952)

Shorter's (1985) second contention was that much of what physicians have to offer is largely the healing power of one person listening to another, with the judicious use of placebos as adjuvant therapy:

Hence, even without many complex theories about psychosomatic mechanisms, [doctors from the 1920s] had enough common sense to realize how much patients benefited from a "good chat." The medical consultation in itself, when conducted in a friendly, leisurely way, can have a curative power. . . . [T]hat curative power is being lost today.

Have physicians lost the skills of therapeutic listening and properly using the mystique of their position? Medical schools in the 1920s and 1930s did not teach listening skills, and faculty did not role-model empathy toward the mentally ill in the clinical training that Watts had described. Again, it is difficult to disprove a hypothesis as intangible as whether doctors of yesteryear were more adept at employing the power of their position as a healing therapy than contemporary physicians are.

In a study conducted in the United Kingdom, a general practitioner again demonstrated that reassuring patients has healing effects (Thomas 1978). Of 470 visits to this practitioner, 200 were for vague symptoms with no obvious, organic cause. The doctor randomized these 200 patients into two groups: One received symptomatic treatment, while the other received no treatment at all. There was no difference between the groups in regard to repeat visits, reports of ongoing symptoms, or recovery rates. The author concluded that many patients presenting with ill-defined symptoms could be safely and effectively treated with reassurance. Numerous articles, editorials, and commentaries repeatedly highlighted the therapeutic effect of a reassuring visit to a trusted physician. In contrast to Shorter, other commentators have argued that today's physicians make even greater use of the curative power of their position than they did in the past.

The objectivity of science upon which progress in therapeutics so heavily depends, paradoxically is suppressed when the physician confronts the patient's need to "take something" and his own urge to "do something." The modern therapist, no less than his colleagues of centuries past, often uses the symbolic power of medication for essentially non-pharmacologic purposes. (Pellegrino 1979)

By the 1960s and 1970s, however, there was substantial societal reaction against the paternal position of authority granted to physicians and outright disgust at the notion that a physician would provide an unwitting and vulnerable patient with a placebo. Notably, this discomfort with the knowing use of placebos was palpable even in the 1930s. Taylor (1954) described a general practitioner's uneasiness and chagrin upon his indoctrination to general practice in 1931:

The dispensary was simple. There was a curtain and some mixtures ready made up in bottles on the shelves. I was instructed to disappear behind the curtain, and to spend not less than two minutes there, and to rattle the bottles frequently and then bring out the bottle of medicine. A book of short stories was provided behind the curtain to distract the mind during the enforced delay.

According to Taylor, this ruse was not common. It demonstrates, however, the tension between the therapeutic use of the physician's position of authority and the societal expectation of informed and empowered patients. In the past, patients and physicians could see, with their own eyes, that the drugs had effects: cathartics (diarrhea), emetics (vomit), diuretics (urine), and sedatives (sleep) gave immediate, demonstrable, physical results. At least the tonic tasted bad. In the 1930s, both physicians and patients understood that the medication did not act specifically against a disease, but as an aid to help bolster the body's intrinsic therapeutic powers and balance. Patients did not expect that the tonics would be effective against specific diseases.

Patient expectations were markedly different at the end of the twentieth century. Vogel and Rosenberg (1979) explained:

Clearly the physician and the great majority of patients no longer share a similar view of the body and the mechanisms which determine health and disease. Differing views of the body and the physician's ability to intervene in its mysterious opacity divide groups and individuals, rather than unifying, as the widely disseminated metaphorical view of body function had still done [in the nineteenth century]. Physicians and patients are no longer bound together by the physiologic activity of the drugs administered. In this sense almost all drugs now act as placebo.

The relationship between physicians and patients has changed. A decline in physicians' listening skills, humanity, or use of their mystique does not explain the change, however. The scientific advances and the technological powers that physicians wield against disease drive a wedge between physicians and patients. The extent to which this wedge must be present in order to provide effective treatment is unclear.

There also has been a backlash from society over the extent to which scientific discovery should dictate social decision-making regarding such moral issues as death and dying, abortion, genetic screening, and cloning, for example. The general public is uncomfortable with the influence that scientists and physicians wield on moral or ethical issues. Patients express concern that physicians are not acting within the patient's moral and ethical framework, but on the basis of a biomedical code unobtainable by the patient (Pellegrino 1979). The patient is always balancing the need to trust, in hope of getting better, with the need to distrust, for fear of losing autonomy. Patients now view what once passed for kindly reassurance or the wink of a placebo as dismissive and paternal.

Other societal changes have significantly contributed to strained patient–physician relationships (Lain Entralgo 1969). One important change is the transformation from a rural–agrarian society to an urban–industrial society. One reason the patient–physician relationship could have developed more easily for people from the 1930s is because they may have shared a person–person relationship outside the medical context. Physicians may have known their patients and their patients' families from the neighborhood or the local church, for example. As communities grew larger and became increasingly urban and industrialized, patients and physicians increasingly met as strangers. Consequently, the physician and patient had to manufacture an artificial relationship, where a natural one had not previously existed. Such a natural relationship still may not develop after a single encounter. One could readily argue that a substantial portion of the perceived degradation in the patient–physician relationship is as much a result of the industrial revolution and urbanization as the biomedical revolution.

Patients and physicians are more mobile today than they were in the past, with multiple career changes and opportunities to move across the city, state, or country with relative ease. Even when one is living in a smaller community, a lifetime relationship with a single physician is rare, and relationships spanning even a decade are becoming more unusual. The physician may be not only a stranger but also a different gender and a different race. He or she may be from a different social stratum, a different culture, a different country, or all of these. If we could transport a nineteenth-century physician from rural America to a twentieth-century urban general medicine practice, this physician would lose much of his legendary power of communication. This is true because these powers emanated from a source within the community, rather than from the physician him- or herself:

In contrast to his professional predecessors, today's physician is no longer the mediator in a generally accepted cultural value system. He deals in a language foreign to the patient; he often is not a member of the same community; he knows little of the patient's lifestyle and family, and the patient knows less about his. When patient and physician meet, stranger meets stranger. The bond between patient and physician is fashioned by the physician's special knowledge, not by his role as a delegated interpreter of a commonly held set of beliefs about health, illness, and their place in human existence. Indeed, in a pluralistic society, the possibility of such a commonly held set of beliefs in increasingly remote. (Vogel and Rosenberg 1979)

Physicians should be aware of the obvious changes in doctor–patient relationship, and educators should train young physicians in listening skills, communication, and meeting the patient as another human being in search of care. There is little evidence, however, that physicians' inherent or innate interpersonal skills have changed.

Shorter's (1985) third contention was that patients before the World War II were simply less likely to perceive their symptoms as reflecting a disease:

People today are sick much more often than before WWII. Americans in the 1920s reported 82 episodes of illness annually per 100 population. The average person was sick less than once per year in the 1920s. In the 1980s, the average person is sick twice per year.

Whereas in the 1920s the average person consulted a doctor 2.9 times per year, in 1981 that figure had risen to 4.6. The explanation is that people are now more willing to define their various symptoms as illnesses, to take care of them, and to report them to investigators.

Shorter's data on episodes of illness came from two different sources for the two different time periods. The methodological differences between the two different sources undermined the comparability of these data, however. One can identify other comparison data that indicated no change in the illness experience of large populations. In a study conducted in London in 1950 among a population of 13,000 people cared for by six physicians, Brotherston and Chave (1956) reported that 76% of the subjects visited a physician at least once during the year of study. The average number of illness episodes reported was 2.3 per person, which was lower than Shorter's figure for the 1920s.

Shorter also reported changes in the number of physician visits per year to provide support for the hypothesis that people are sick more often today than they were in the past. For the 1980s, he quoted an average of 4.6 physician visits per year. However, as Shorter himself noted, this figure had been stable, as reported by the National Center for Health Statistics, as far back as 1960. Thus, Shorter was suggesting that the increased frequency of sickness episodes happened sometime before 1960. Even in 1950, however, the rate was about the same: The Health Insurance Plan of Greater New York showed a rate of five physician visits per year per enrollee, based on data from 235,000 people (Baehr 1950).

Another explanation for the difference that Shorter reported is based on a change in occupational law and employer's obligations that occurred between the two periods. In the earlier period, people did not visit the doctor as often because their work would not allow it. There is little evidence to suggest a change in utilization rates at least as far back as 1950. Furthermore, rates of patients visiting doctors have varied across studies. John Fry (1966) reviewed data on patient visits, as reported by three different governmental entities involved with the United Kingdom's National Health Service during 1936–1938. He found reported rates of 5.0, 3.6, and 5.1 visits per person per year, respectively. In Fry's own study conducted in 1949, the rate was 3.8 per person and 75% of his registered patients consulted him that year (Fry 1952). Brotherston and Chave (1956) reviewed rates reported by various investigators from 1950 to 1955 and reported figures ranging from 2.9 to 7.0 visits per person per year.

Shorter's comparisons also failed to consider changes in access to care over the period of inquiry. In both the United Kingdom and the United States, government programs improved access to care for substantial segments of the population. There is evidence that those who had poor access before these programs were instituted increased their visit rates after they began (Hollingsworth 1986). There can be little doubt that patients' help-seeking behaviors and expectations have changed. People rarely sought help for diphtheria and tuberculosis in the 1990s, and people in the 1940s didn't necessarily present with emotional symptoms by using the word "depression." Changes in help-seeking behaviors largely have resulted from changes in the patterns of disease, concepts of disease, treatment choices, and access. The existing research findings do not support a systematic overinterpretation of symptoms by late-twentieth-century patients.

Multiple, systematic studies over the past half-century have provided an accurate picture of the primary-care environment and primary-care physicians. When faced with current problems, many people find it appealing to reminisce about the advantages of yesteryear. Depression is an illness that may be sensitive to the health of the patient–physician relationship. Because of this, some analysts have contended that primary care physicians' declining skills explain an overreliance on medication, poor outcomes, excess costs, and dissatisfaction.

Primary care is a remarkably complex arena in which to practice medicine. Ferris, writing in 1967, described the general practitioner's destiny as follows:

Every day from Monday to Friday, 24,000 general practitioners see close to a million people. . . . They meet all the emotions, from fright to lust. In a year an average practice will have 20 to 30 deaths and rather more births. The doctor will be presented with thousands of coughs and colds and skin disorders, a lot of indigestion, some ulcers, a little madness and much private misery, many anemias and waxed-up ears, a few cancers and heart attacks, a trace of acute appendicitis and tuberculosis, a divorce, a sprinkling of alcoholics and a half-dozen problem families. A third to half of all the illness he sees may be "neurotic" in origin. . . . Clinically, he will be a clever man if he can see the wood for the trees.

Summary

It is imperative that we accurately depict both the merits and demerits of medical practice in the twentieth century so that we can map out how the treatment model for depression has changed—if it has changed at all. The research we have presented in this chapter supports our view that the basic constitution, dedication, interpersonal talents, work capacity, and humanity of general practitioners have changed little, if at all, over the past half-century. Physical facilities and therapeutic choices at mid-century were clearly much more limited, if not deplorable, by today's standards. There is little evidence to suggest that primary-care physicians' visits were longer or more focused on listening, empathy, or counseling than they are today.

There is ample evidence that these physicians were just as likely to prescribe symptomatic, sedating, or psychoactive medications. On one hand, a cynic might view this argument with the pessimistic conclusion that primary care has always been in a state of semi-chaos, reflecting a poor knowledge base and ineffective patient–physician communication. On the other hand, one could contend that, even in the face of enormous scientific and cultural changes, primary care has been able to adapt its service and quality to keep pace with societal demands. We found no evidence to support the myth of the "old-time doctor" and no evidence that current doctors suffer from a systematic decline in professionalism.

We also found no evidence to support the contention of measurable changes in patients' basic constitution, pain tolerance, or rates of emotional distress. In addition, rates of patients' visits to physicians have changed very little over the past half-century, including rates of patients' visits for emotional symptoms. This suggests that patients today are not more likely to complain than they were in the past. This raises the question of why emotional symptoms have not declined, however. With all of the improvements in public health during the past half-century and with all of the improvements in specific treatments for depression, why are emotional symptoms still so prevalent?

At mid-century, society regarded the deficiencies of primary care as unacceptable. Primary care had as many issues regarding the quality and efficiency of care for medical disorders as it did about emotional disorders. It had not kept pace with the therapeutic revolution, and it had to change. The forces that led to this critical system redesign are important to our examining the leadership versus followship role of primary care. The next chapter describes how the United Kingdom and the United States redesigned primary care.

5

PRIMARY CARE IN CRISIS

The Common Dilemma

In a presidential address to the American Medical Association, W. L. Bierring (1934) reminded his audience of society's influence on the delivery of health care:

Since the turn of the century, man's environment has changed, largely as a result of the expansion of his control over physical forces, as in the growth of speed, the elimination of time and space, and the enlargement of the dominion of man's skill and knowledge. This new environment has however not produced a new society, and in some respects the individual units of society have not kept pace with the changing world.

Although this commentary resonates with the current state of health-care affairs, Bierring delivered this presidential address in 1934. He went on to predict that primary care would be the bedrock of a rational American health-care system, fulfill the potential of preventive health care, influence medical science in its societal debates, and assuage society's ambivalence toward science. Many of his predictions were remarkably prescient. While a comprehensive evaluation of the societal changes occurring in Britain and America during the past 50 years is beyond the scope of this book, it is necessary to understand the political and social climate of primary care throughout this period. Chapters 2–4 depicted primary care at mid-century; this chapter describes changes in the health-care delivery systems in the United States and the United Kingdom over the past half-century.

Changes in the larger system of primary care explain much about our current approach to emotional disorders.

Until World War II, a British and an American citizen seeking care from a general practitioner in their respective societies would have been seeking care in similar health-care systems. As late as 1950, medical-care expenditures as a percentage of gross national product were similar in the United Kingdom and the United States at 4.1% and 4.6%, respectively (Hollingsworth 1986). Although England had national health insurance as early as 1913, the program only provided access to medical care to low-income workers.

In the 1950s and 1960s, multiple analysts described general practitioners as discontented, isolated, and demoralized. Indeed, some authorities expressed concern that the entire field might disappear. Between 1930 and 1960, the number of general-practice physicians in the United States declined from 90 per 100,000 population to fewer than 40 (Huntley 1963). Between 1952 and 1965, the number of general practitioners working in solo practices fell from 43% to 24%, and the number of medical students choosing a career in general practice plummeted. Haggerty (1963) cited lower prestige, less money, less research activity, fewer hospital privileges, and time pressures as the reasons for the declining number of medical students interested in pursuing careers in general medicine. McWhinney (1966), writing in the *Lancet*, asked: Why is the general practitioner disappearing?

I asked this question many times and usually got the same answers. Certainly not for lack of reward. American general practitioners can earn a good income, often better than some specialists. Medical students are shunning general practice because it lacks academic prestige.

Some analysts cited income and prestige disparities between generalists and specialists, hospitals' preference for specialists, the loss of practice autonomy, or the general practitioner's failure to understand his or her clinical limitations as reasons for the decline. Others cited the public's growing fascination with technology and hospital-based medicine.

Either policy makers exaggerated the risk of primary care's collapse, or its reorganization over the following decade prevented its fall—or both. In reality, the notion that general practice is a dying profession is at least 100 years old. In 1946, speaking before the Section on the General Practice of Medicine at the 95th Annual Session of the American Medical Association, William M. Johnson reflected:

Some of you are old enough to remember that after the First World War there was a similar trend toward specialism. Then, as now, experts published obituary notices for the family doctor. Long before World War I—in 1902—Sir William Osler told the Canadian Medical Association that "it is amusing to read and hear of the passing of the family physician."

Johnson agreed, however, that general practice had important problems. The advances in medical science and changing societal expectations demanded that general practice, on both sides of the Atlantic, transform itself. However, the course of action pursued on the two sides of the Atlantic proved to be fundamentally different.

After World War II, both the British and American health-care systems began to move away from the model of general practice that had been relatively constant since the late nineteenth century. Because of society's role in shaping health-care, the British and American health care systems diverged in their approach to "the common dilemma": that the public and professional "wants" will always be greater than politically defined "needs," which in turn will always be greater than the national "resources" for health care (Fry and Horder 1994).

The British Response

In the July 3, 1948, issue of the *British Medical Journal*, Aneurin Bevan, the Minister of Health and one of the principal architects of the National Health Service, wrote an open letter to the medical profession:

On July 5 there is no reason why the whole of the doctor–patient relationship should not be freed from what most of us feel should be irrelevant to it, the money factor, the collection of fees or the thinking how to pay fees—an aspect of practice already distasteful to many practitioners. Yet it has been vital, if this is to be the new situation, to see that it did not carry with it either any discouragement of professional and scientific freedom or any unfair worsening of a doctor's material livelihood.

The picture I have always visualized is one, not of "panel doctoring" for the less well off, not of anything charitable or demeaning, but rather of a nation deciding to make health-care easier and more effective by pooling its resources.

Six months earlier, in January 1948, in a referendum taken by the British Medical Association, 84% of the general practitioners had voted against initiating the National Health Service. Despite this opposition, on July 5, 1948, the United Kingdom instituted the National Health Service, which divided its funds into three "pots": hospital care, general-practice care, and social services (Bevan 1948). General practitioners received a capitation payment, which depended on the number and characteristics of their assigned patients. List sizes, or the number of patients assigned to each general practitioner, ranged from 2000 to 4000. Although there were plans to devote funding toward improving the general practitioners' offices, in the first decade, most of the funds went to hospitals (Webster 1988). Thus, British general practice stagnated in the 1950s and 1960s. Webster commented that "in the first phase of the National Health Service . . . it is difficult to avoid the conclusion that general medical practice was treated by the health departments as a receding backwater." The U.K. government's original intent, however, was to design a universal health-care system with general practice as the foundation. One of its accomplishments during this early period of redesigning primary care was a concerted attempt to effect a rational and equitable distribution of general practitioners throughout the country.

Despite considerable debate and temporizing measures to help general practice, little change occurred at a public policy level for 20 years. In 1964, the British Medical Association proposed a mass resignation of general practitioners from the National Health Service and requested undated letters of resignation from all member general practitioners (Fry 1988). In addition, general practitioners prepared to organize an independent health service (General Medical Services Committee 1965). The American Medical Association, in the thick of a debate about national health insurance in the United States at the same time, was aware of this professional discontent in Britain.

Relief for British general practitioners came in 1966, when the National Health Service implemented the Family Doctor Charter, which contained provisions to change how much the government paid general practitioners, including not only an increase in capitation rates but also an allowance for additional fees for certain services. In other words, a proportion of the general practitioners' practices became fee-for-service. The Family Doctor Charter also provided funding for continuing medical education and practice expenses, including money for ancillary staff and facility improvements. The new capital enabled many general practitioners to hire receptionists, clerical staff, and nurses; as a result, more practices were able to adopt appointment systems and improve medical record keeping.

These changes accelerated the development of larger group practices. Larger practices enabled physicians to develop on-call rotations and more predictable daily schedules. In the following decade, debate and legislation led general practice to be officially recognized as a medical specialty, as well as to improvements in general practitioners' vocational training. Many leaders in British general practice consider this charter to be the main reason for the renaissance in general practice in the United Kingdom. In addition, the Family Doctor Charter reiterated and reinvigorated the idea that general practitioners were the cornerstone of the National Health System.

Many evolutionary changes in how the British health-care system was administered occurred in the 1970s. However, a substantial reorganization of the National Health Service took place in 1974, when the British government established Community Health Councils. As part of this reorganization, Britain allocated new funds to develop Health Centers, which housed small groups of general practitioners, as well as nurses, social workers, public health officials, and other allied health professionals. The goals of these centers were to support a team approach to primary care and community outreach and to improve collaboration between general practitioners and specialists (Webster 1988). By 1986, the number of British general practitioners in solo practices fell from 43% to 11%. By the 1980s, through coalescence into group practices and adding ancillary staff, the typical practice "team" encompassed 30 people or more (Fry 1988). Public policy officials still debate the success of the 1974 reorganization, but there is some evidence that the changes improved communication and allocation of resources among hospitals, general practice, and public health. Unfortunately, by the late 1970s, concerns about the rate of increase in the cost of the National Health Service began playing a larger part in shaping health-care policy. Also, with improvements in organizing practices, public health officials could monitor quality of care because there was a more extensive infrastructure for these activities.

In 1964, the care provided in the National Health Service satisfied most patients, even though many aspects of the primary care system were demonstrably substandard. Cartwright and Marshall (1965) wrote that "behind the satisfaction of most patients there lies an uncritical acceptance and lack of discrimination which is conducive to stagnation and apathy." In 1977, Ann Cartwright repeated her study of patient satisfaction, which she had originally conducted in 1964 (Cartwright and Anderson 1981). The study assessed the influence of the many changes in the system of general-practice health care over the previous decade. As expected, she documented dramatic changes in the physical facilities that were consistent with the incentives that the Family Doctor Charter had provided. More physicians were in group practices; many more of their premises were purposefully built; more were employing receptionists, nurses, and clerical staff; and more were using appointment systems. Waiting times had decreased, and doctors spent less time on call. Contrary to expectations, however, Cartwright did not find improvements in patients' and physicians' attitudes.

Both patients and physicians reported that patients were more knowledgeable about health issues than they had been a decade earlier. There were no changes in physician satisfaction, however. In 1964, some 56% of physicians reported that at least one-quarter of their patient visits were for trivial reasons; in 1977, at 50%, this figure had hardly changed (Cartwright and Anderson 1981). Either the immense changes in the structure and process of care were irrelevant to patients' and physicians' attitudes, or expectations had increased in parallel with improvements.

In the early 1990s, increasingly motivated by cost concerns, the National Health Service again experienced a fundamental reorganization. The goal of the change was to introduce "market influences" into the British Health Care system in order to increase efficiency, improve quality, and decrease costs through competition. Capitation payments grew substantially, and general practitioners became the "purchasers" of health care for their panel of patients. The National Health Insurance introduced "budget-holding," which allowed the regional Family Health Service Authorities to purchase specialist care for their patients from either the National Health Service or private sources. From a patient's perspective, this placed the physician in a position of potential conflict of interest:

The rationing of health care had always been a part of the general practitioner's work, but had previously been implied rather than stated. Now, particularly in fund-holding practice, and in the tension between fund-holding and non-fund-holding, the general practitioner's ethical duty to advocate justice for the individual patient became strained by the additional ethical duty to achieve distributive justice for the community. (Marinker 1998)

The 1990s reforms also led to more oversight of certain aspects of medical performance, such as practice guidelines, targets for preventive health care, and health education. The National Health Service required general practitioners to provide specified services and encouraged innovation in care. For example, groups of general practitioners might develop unique features in team care, such as "specialized" general practice, or creative approaches to practice design and purchasing arrangements.

These changes increased the general practitioners' administrative and team-leadership roles, which included direct patient care, disease management, preventive health, and purchasing secondary care (Bosanquet and Salisbury 1998). In addition, the National Health Service designed other policies to enhance patient rights, in terms of both obtaining health care and participating in policy development. The "Patient's Charter," for example, encouraged providers to report their performance measures, such as waiting times for surgery, so that patients could make informed choices among providers.

There are still many concerns about the National Health Service and the degree to which its focus on primary care has truly resulted in the continuity of care (Williamson 1964; Watkin 1978; Honigsbaum 1979; Hart 1994). Regardless of current judgments about the National Health System's strengths, the primary-care environment in the United Kingdom has passed through several cycles of crisis and reorganization over the past half-century, which has affected both help-seeking and treatments for emotional disorders.

The American Response

The United States has experienced multiple failed attempts to enact a national health policy. Most of these efforts have involved legislation for compulsory health insurance, with the premiums to be paid through taxes or payroll deductions. Opponents have defeated each of these attempts beginning as early as 1916 and including a substantial, organized, political effort nearly every decade since that time. Even in 1935, in a political climate that resulted in the Social Security Act, opponents defeated universal health insurance. The Social Security Act provided financial support for unemployment, retirement income, and public assistance for certain groups, but it did not provide for their health insurance. In almost all prior attempts, the likelihood of enacting national health insurance appeared imminent just before it faded away (Numbers 1979; Starr 1982; Stevens 1998). At the beginning of the twenty-first century, the United States remained one of the few established market economies with no nationally organized, funded health-care system.

Multiple factors figured into the defeats of prior efforts to establish national health insurance, and each defeat reflected the various societal concerns and special interests of the particular era during which it was proposed (Starr 1982;

Skocpol 1996; Stevens 1998). However, one common theme in these defeats has been a societal concern that federal government control and management of health care were affronts to the American ideal of personal liberty. In 1946, delivering the Presidential Address at the 95th Annual Session of the American Medical Association just after the end of World War II, H. H. Shoulders exemplified the fervor of this sentiment:

> The issue before the American people is becoming more clearly defined and in brief it is this: Shall patients and doctors retain their freedom of judgment in this matter of medical care or shall this freedom be surrendered to a federal bureaucracy?
>
> Not long ago our freedom was challenged by foes from without. That challenge has been met and repelled. A challenge, no less definite, has been made by the foes of freedom from within. The question is: Shall we surrender, shall we abandon the principles that have made the profession and the nation great?

The legislation to which Shoulders referred would have allowed all licensed physicians in the United States to act as a first point of contact for care. A physician in the federal government, however, would have been responsible for determining which physicians could act as specialists. The focus of health care would have rested with primary-care physicians, and patients would not have had the right to seek specialist care unless their physicians referred them. The legislation was similar in many ways to the proposed National Health Service, which was under debate in the United Kingdom at the same time.

Of particular importance to successfully opposing national health insurance has been special interests groups' access to financing and expertise in working within the political system (Starr 1982). Economic interests have always played a role in shaping health-care policy. Even in those countries with a national health system, economic interests have been a driving force:

> We associate health insurance with the financing of medical care, but its original function was primarily income stabilization. . . . Governmental programs were originally conceived as a means of maintaining the incomes, productive effort, and political allegiance of the working class. (Starr 1982)

Besides the commonly noted opponents, such as insurance companies, Starr (1982) pointed out that other special interest groups were willing to bargain for their own gains in return for opposing or remaining silent on health care reform:

> The hospitals sought relief through aid for construction, and the medical schools through aid for research. The culmination of the piecemeal approach was categorical legislation on behalf of constituencies organized around specific diseases, such as cancer and heart disease. The opposition to compulsory insurance did not prevent a steady growth in state intervention in medical care. Government financing increased, but it was channeled into avenues that did not, at least immediately, threaten professional sovereignty.

In a review of the most recent attempts at health care reform, Skocpol (1996) reported that, in 1958, over 70% of Americans responded that "always or most of the time" they could trust the federal government to do what was right. By 1994, however, fewer than 20% of Americans endorsed this statement. Although it is sometimes easy to blame American politicians or other special interest groups, Skocpol aptly described the complexity of the U.S. political process:

> We should not allow our attention to be directed away from the nation's major institutions—its government, mass media, political parties, and health care and economic enterprises. These were the arenas within which our leaders—not just those in the Clinton administration but also corporate leaders, journalists, health care providers, and Democrats and Republicans in Congress and beyond—defined their goals and maneuvered in relation to each other. Within and at the intersection of these institutions, America's leaders failed to come up with reasonable ways to address pressing national concerns about the financing of health care for everyone.

One result of the lack of a national health system is the lack of an authoritative mandate affirming primary care as the foundation of medical care in the United States. Depending on their ability to pay, Americans can seek "first-contact" care from a plastic surgeon or a cardiologist as readily as they can from a general practitioner. The absence of a defined role for general practice and the proliferation of specialists in the postwar period have resulted in a crisis of purpose for general practitioners in the United States. General practitioners fought not only to keep government out of their practices but also to keep specialists from subverting their patients and prestige, the hospitals from removing their hospital privileges, and advancements in medical sciences from overwhelming their model of care (Stevens 1998).

Between 1950 and 1965, the main mechanism for financing medical care in the United States was private health insurance. Employees obtained this insurance through their employers, and employers wielded collective bargaining power over the cost of care. In 1958, two-thirds of Americans had insurance coverage for hospital costs. Private health insurance, however, paid less than 25% of the total per capita health-care expenditures (Numbers 1979). People with jobs and those with higher incomes were the most likely to have health insurance (Starr 1982). Also, veterans were eligible for care in an expanding Veterans Affairs health-care system that the federal government financed and organized. By 1966, at least 81% of the civilian population had some hospital benefits (Stevens 1998). During this period, primary-care physicians received payment almost entirely in a fee-for-service arrangement. Physicians' average incomes rose substantially, and the entire medical industry enjoyed an enormous expansion. In addition, medical research experienced a huge expansion in funding. For example, the National Institutes of Health's budget increased from $4 million in 1947 to $400 million in 1960. Despite huge expenditures on individual fragments of a health-care system, large segments of the American population remained uninsured, including many of its most vulnerable citizens.

In 1965, legislators enacted the Medicare and Medicaid programs. Medicare is a federally administered program that provides hospital insurance for older Americans and a government-subsidized voluntary insurance to pay for physician's bills. Medicaid provides poor Americans with health insurance. Individual states administer the Medicaid program, setting the eligibility requirements and coverage limits. At mid-century, American primary-care physicians complained about their falling professional prestige, much like their British counterparts. In the spirit of the aphorism "a rising tide raises all ships," the rising income of American general practitioners and their relative professional autonomy offset this disquiet. Thus, although a primary-care physician might be sending bills to private insurance companies, Medicare, Medicaid, and even the Veterans Administration, they were receiving payment.

This period of growing authority, economic prosperity, and autonomy for the American medical establishment began to erode in the 1970s, as the costs of medical care soared. Throughout the 1970s and 1980s, debate regarding how to keep these growing costs in check resulted in much regulatory legislation, but no concerted or effective effort to initiate a national health system. From the primary-care physician's perspective, this was a period of increasing bureaucratic interference, administrative duties, paperwork, and antagonism with patients. Also, during this period, most segments of the health-care industry came under increasing regulatory control. Legislation focused on curbing costs and redirected the financial incentives from supporting doing more to doing less. This led to legislation that stimulated the growth of health maintenance organizations (HMOs) as one mechanism to provide incentives intended to promote health rather than the delivery of health care.

Payers provide HMOs with a capitated payment to deliver health care to a defined population. Preferred Provider Organizations (PPOs), which provide care to groups of people for a discounted fee and provide oversight on the use of services, also began during this period. In the 1970s, fewer than 5% of the American population were enrolled in an HMO, but by the 1980s, about 25% of Americans participated in an HMO or PPO. Even in the 1980s, however, most of primary-care physicians' income continued to come from fee-for-service care.

The idea of managed competition appeared in the U.S. health-care industry in the mid-1980s, and it has driven health-care policy for most of the last two decades. Proponents argue that if providers compete against each other on value to the informed consumer, then the quality of care will improve and costs will decline. With this logic, more successful providers will drive less-efficient providers out of the market. There is some evidence that this occurred in the United States in the 1990s, when many smaller hospitals, HMOs, and insurance schemes folded. Also, many hospitals merged in an attempt to reduce the duplication of services and improve efficiencies. An increasing number of Americans are now receiving health care in some type of managed-care setting. As many as 50% of workers who participate in a health-care plan provided by their employer now participate in a managed-care program rather than a fee-for-service arrangement (Rothman 1997).

In an effort to further reduce costs and improve quality, the larger managed-care organizations and the federal government have developed clinical-practice guidelines, regulations on using technology, and quality-performance indicators. Access to specialist services has come under increasing control and, especially in areas dominated by managed-care organizations, primary-care physicians have been in demand. All of the federally funded programs, including Medicare, Medicaid, and the Veterans Affairs hospitals, have endorsed the principles of managed competition.

While experts accept that these ostensibly "market-driven" changes have reduced the growth of health-care expenditures, the magnitude of this reduction is unclear. Also, it is very difficult to assess the effect of these changes on the quality of care. There is no question that these changes have reduced the primary-care practitioner's autonomy, brought greater scrutiny of his or her practice patterns, and moved a greater percentage of his or her patients out of fee-for-service arrangements. Notably, policy makers did not design any of these developments to address the issue of the uninsured population specifically. Thus, patients with emotional symptoms presenting to primary-care providers in the United States will have different access, hassles, and cost of care, depending on their insurer or lack of one.

Which Primary Care System Is the Best?

After 50 years of advances in medical science, different political and societal pressures, and divergent paths in dealing with "the common dilemma," how different are the health-care systems in the United States and the United Kingdom? In this section we summarize comparisons of the two systems as reported by several authors (Starfield 1991, 1992; Fry and Horder 1994; Fry et al. 1995; Horder 1998). The most glaring difference is cost. Total health-care expenditures in the United States in 1997 were nearly $1 trillion for a population of approximately 270 million; per capita health-care expenditures were $3925 (Kramarow et al. 1999). The United States accounts for about 5% of the world's population but consumes about 40% of the global health-care resources (Fry et al. 1995). Between 1960 and 1990, U.S. health-care expenditures as a percentage of gross domestic product rose from 5.1% to 13.5%. Payment for about 42% of health-care costs come from public funds and the remainder from private funds. Administrative costs in the United States account for 20% of the health-care budget (Fry and Horder 1994). Per capita expenditures for medications are about $165.

In comparison, the total health-care expenditures in the United Kingdom in 1997 were about $80 billion for a population of approximately 59 million; thus per capita health-care expenditures were $1347 (Kramarow et al. 1999). Between

1960 and 1990, health-care expenditures as a percentage of gross domestic product rose from 3.9% to 6.7%. Payments for about 85% of health-care costs come from public funds. Administrative costs in the United Kingdom are about 6% of the total health-care budget (Fry and Horder 1994). Per capita expenditures for medications are $96. Thus, the U.S. population is more than 4.5 times larger than the U.K.'s population, but its total health-care expenditures are about 12 times greater. The United States spends nearly 3 times more per person for health care than the United Kingdom does.

Despite substantial differences in expenditures, the primary health measures of the two nations are equivalent, and both have improved since mid-century (Hollingsworth 1986; Fry and Horder 1994). Life expectancy at birth in the United States is 72.8 years for males and 79.5 years for females; there are 9 deaths per year per 1000 population; and the infant mortality rate is 7 per 1000 live births. C omparatively, life expectancy at birth in the United Kingdom is 74 years for males and 79 years for females; there are 11 deaths per year per 1000 population; and the infant mortality rate is 6 per 1000 live births.

In their comparison of the primary health systems in 12 different industrialized nations, including the United States and the United Kingdom, Fry and Horder (1994) noted:

It was remarkable that in all countries the clinical and social problems dealt with by the primary health care workers were similar. The common conditions encountered were a mix of minor ailments, serious diseases and chronic disorders and social issues and care of the dying. Generally they were also managed in similar ways clinically and socially. The health systems differed. Administrative structures depended on sources of funding, levels of managerial and executive decentralization, and particularly on the ways in which physicians were paid, with what incentives and reward. Yet, paradoxically, in spite of these quite major differences, the crude outcomes in terms of health indices were similar.

It is not possible to adjudge one health-care system as better than another among the major industrialized nations based on health-care outcomes. In general, Americans spend more and express more dissatisfaction with their health-care system than do citizens of any other nation (Blendon et al. 1990). Americans also have higher expectations for care, expect to spend more for care, and have a greater distrust of federal control of the health-care system (Blendon et al. 1995). While U.S. physicians report significant problems with patient access to care, physicians in countries with universal coverage report greater problems with nursing shortages and access to well-equipped facilities and sophisticated medical technology (Blendon et al. 1993). In a recent study of public satisfaction with care across five countries, including the United States and the United Kingdom, in no country were most people satisfied with their health-care system. In countries with universal coverage, public discontent centered on inadequate spending, administration, and waiting times. In the United States, the public was primarily concerned with financial barriers to care (Donelan et al. 1999).

One posited reason why health outcomes are so similar is that the health-care system is not the only determinant of health. Other determinants—such as lifestyle, self-care behaviors, personal preferences, education, income, and socioeconomic status—are equally important (Hollingsworth 1986; Wilkinson 1992, 1999). For example, Starfield (1992) found that the United States had perhaps the most poorly organized primary health-care system of the various countries studied and that some key indicators of the process, outcomes, and satisfaction with care reflected inadequacies in primary care (Starfield 1991). In contrast, the United Kingdom scored well on measures related to the organization of primary health care, but there was poor concordance with key health indicators and public satisfaction. She suggested that "the lack of concordance in the ratings in the United Kingdom may be a result of low expenditures for other social services and public education in that country."

How Does the System of Care Affect the Process of Care?

Only a few studies have examined the differences in the philosophy and process of care between the United States and the United Kingdom (Mechanic 1972; Marsh et al. 1976; Hull 1981). Mechanic (1972) completed an extensive study of the practice patterns of primary-care physicians in the two countries and found marked differences in the content of their clinical encounters. Overall, British general practitioners provided a much broader range of services than primary-care providers in the United States did. The researchers viewed some of these services, such as performing minor surgical procedures, as appropriate to the providers' skills. They found that less-trained providers could provide many other services. In addition, while U.S. general practices were narrower, these physicians tended to complete more extensive clinical evaluations, spent more time with patients, and collaborated more with their specialist colleagues. Mechanic also reported that British general practitioners were more professionally isolated and disillusioned than their U.S. counterparts.

Marsh and colleagues (1976) also reported a study of differences in practice styles between British and American general practitioners. These investigators reported that British physicians spent more time and placed more diagnostic emphasis on the patient's history, whereas U.S. physicians completed more thorough physical examinations and were more likely to complete specific components of the physical examination related to preventive health, such as blood pressure monitoring. The U.S. physicians were much more likely to order diagnostic testing, such as routine blood tests, radiographs, and electrocardiograms. British physicians were more likely to request specialty consultations and to diagnose patients with emotional disorders, although both groups of physicians were equally likely to prescribe psychoactive medications. The authors opined that American patients "expected" a physical examination and diagnostic testing, while British patients did not. They also suggested that British patients were more willing than American patients to accept a psychiatric diagnosis without an extensive search for an organic illness.

Numerous authors have written about the importance of culture on both help-seeking behaviors and the provision of health care, suggesting that there are complex interactions among society, the health system, help-seeking behaviors, and physicians' practice patterns. Are the health systems different because of patients' expectations and providers' practice styles, or have patients' expectations and providers' practice styles been the main force in determining the structure of the respective health-care systems? Do providers' practice styles drive patients' expectations, or vice versa? History and prior research would suggest that these effects are interactive and that multiple factors outside of the health-care system also play a role in determining the structure, process, and outcomes of care.

Summary

There are fundamental differences in the history and design of the health-care systems in the United States and the United Kingdom. The most obvious difference relates to overall costs. In terms of major indices like mortality, the increased expenditures in the United States have not been accompanied by important advantages in health-care outcomes. For individual diseases, such as breast cancer or coronary artery disease, the United States has netted better outcomes. Among certain racial or socioeconomic groups, however, health outcomes in the United States are poorer than they are in the United Kingdom.

Besides expenditures, differences in the foundation of primary care may be the greatest design contrast. The National Health Service recognizes primary-care physicians as the bedrock of its health-care system and as the first point of contact. The cost of primary care is not a barrier for citizens in the United Kingdom. Unfortunately, U.K. patients with fewer socioeconomic resources continue to have poorer outcomes, even with the United Kingdom's easier access to care. Clearly, there are other important determinants of health outcomes beyond the design of the formal health-care system. Thus, when comparing outcomes between the two countries, the answers differ, depending on which group of citizens, diseases, or outcomes we choose to investigate.

In some respects, the structural features of the two systems have become increasingly similar over the past 60 years. For example, the U.S. Department of Health and Human Services reports that 77 million Americans are enrolled in HMOs, compared with approximately 60 million Britons cared for in the National Health Service. In addition, more than 70 million Americans are enrolled in Medicare and Medicaid programs (Kramarow et al. 1999). In 1993, more than 6 million Britons (more than 10% of the population) held private medical insurance. Both countries have moved toward managed competition as a mechanism to reduce costs and have embraced clinical practice guidelines and performance indicators to improve quality. Both countries also encourage patients' greater participation in health-care decisions and self-care.

Given what we know about the two health-care systems and about the nature of current treatment recommendations for emotional disorders, one would expect that a system such as that available in the United Kingdom would lead to better outcomes for patients with depression. Reduced financial barriers to medical care and a system that supports stronger patient–provider relationships should result in better treatment rates. In Chapter 10, we explore how the two countries compare in their treatment outcomes for emotional disorders.

Part II

ORIGINS OF THE CURRENT
TREATMENT MODEL
FOR DEPRESSION

6

FROM WORLD WAR TO MAGIC BULLETS
TO MASS STRATEGY

Thus far, we have presented evidence that most people who seek medical care for emotional disorders turn to primary-care physicians rather than to psychiatrists. We also presented evidence that society, cultural values, and the design of health-care systems influence how and when people decide to seek care for emotional disorders and how doctors treat patients with emotional disorders. Primary-care doctors and patients have changed much less than our labels and treatments for depression would suggest, and there has been little change in the rate at which people seek care for emotional disorders. This chapter serves as a bridge from the story of primary care to the story of psychiatry. Before turning to the history of how psychiatrists treat severe mental illness in Chapter 7, this chapter describes the major changes in how generalists treat medical diseases.

A history of innovations in psychiatry must be told in the context of the history of innovations in the prevention and treatment of medical illnesses. Discoveries in other areas of medical science prepared the way for discoveries in psychiatry and changed the epidemiology of medical illness seen in primary care, which consequently influenced the health-care delivery system and altered the demands on primary-care physicians. As a result of these changes, there was a shift from a primary-care model that focused on acute infectious diseases in individual patients to a model that emphasized managing or preventing chronic diseases in communities. Before describing the history of therapeutics for depression, we first provide a brief history of discoveries in medical therapeutics. These discoveries completely changed the spectrum of illness, as well as primary care doctors' responsibilities and daily lives.

The Exigencies of War

Located in St. Paul's Cathedral in London, the Golden Book is a roll of honor containing the names of the men and women commemorated in the cathedral's American Memorial Chapel. Shortly after World War II, General Dwight D. Eisenhower made the following dedication in the Golden Book:

All who shall hereafter live in freedom will be here reminded that to these men and their comrades we owe a debt to be paid with grateful remembrance of their sacrifice and with high resolve that the cause for which they died shall live eternally.

This dedication is inscribed in stone on the Wall of the Missing at the American Military Cemetery, the only permanent American World War II cemetery in the United Kingdom, which is located on the outskirts of Cambridge. The Wall of the Missing is nearly 500 feet long and contains the names of over 5000 service personnel missing in action or buried at sea.

The county of Cambridgeshire surrounding Cambridge contains expansive areas of flat land that were ideal for the large airfields that heavy bombers required. Consequently, this county was the site of more than 25 airfields during World War II. Although these airfields played a decisive role in the Allied victory, the human costs were enormous. During the countless bombing sorties from these airfields over a five-year period, the Royal Air Force lost 55,500 personnel, and the United States lost 43,000 (Smith 1997). Cambridge thus became a favorite destination of British and American aviators, who were searching for a brief relief from the stresses of war. On the ceiling of the Eagle, a pub that sits among the buildings and colleges of Cambridge University, some of these aviators signed their names using smoke from cigarette lighters and candles. These ephemeral gestures of young men facing the prospect of death in the service of their country remain visible more than 50 years later.

At Oxford during World War II, Florey and Chain were studying the clinical applications of penicillin, while in the United States, Waksman was discovering the properties of streptomycin that would lead to successful treatments for tuberculosis. Still other British and American scientists were working on synthesizing anti-malarial compounds, mechanisms to combat cardiovascular shock, innovations in trauma surgery, anesthesia, and improvements in systems design for emergency medicine. With the same sense of urgency with which British and American civilians were building bombers and British and American aviators were fighting in the skies over Europe, British and American scientists were studying new therapies to keep the military forces healthy, including treatment for combat fatigue. These therapies not only changed the course of acute illnesses for countless people during the war, but they also set the stage for a paradigm of discovery for medical therapeutics that continues today. The discovery and manufacture of penicillin is the prototype in this new system of science. We spend some time describing the story of penicillin because it set the stage for our model of medical research for the last half-century.

The story of penicillin is compelling not only because it set off a therapeutic revolution but also because it contains four recurring themes in the discovery of psychotherapeutics. The first theme demonstrates that bringing a discovery from its inception to clinical application is not the province of a single scientist. Instead, breakthroughs and revolutions result from the incremental work of teams of scientists, often followed by collaborations among academia, government, and industry to move the discovery out of the laboratory toward practical application.

The second theme shows our faith in the existence of a magic bullet awaiting elucidation for the cure of a specific disease. Although experts denounced the promise of magic bullets as science fiction when Paul Ehrlich first introduced them in 1906 (Weatherall 1990), his idea was prophetic:

If we picture an organism as infected by a certain species of bacterium, it will obviously be easy to effect a cure if substances have been discovered which have an exclusive affinity for the bacteria and act deleteriously or lethally on these, and on these alone, while at the same time, they possess no affinity whatever for the normal constituents of the body and cannot therefore have the least harmful or other effect on that body. Such substances would then be able to exert their final action exclusively on the parasite harbored within the organism and would represent, so to speak, magic bullets which seek their target of their own accord. (Himmelwert 1960)

We now expect drugs that we can easily ingest without side effects that will halt or prevent an infectious agent with precise specificity. More important for our story, we also expect that there will be magic bullets for noninfectious diseases. Throughout the nineteenth century and through the first half of the twentieth century, physicians prescribed nonspecific treatments that they believed would help patients regain their equilibrium through general and visible measures. These measures promised to strengthen the patient's constitution, augmenting his or her own inherent homeostatic mechanisms. The idea was that illness could be cured by strengthening the host rather than by weakening an invader. By the mid-twentieth century, we replaced this framework with an understanding that specific invaders or imbalances cause illness (Pellegrino 1979).

The third theme in this magic bullet paradigm is that scientists, policy makers, and society became convinced that we could solve any problem, regardless of its complexity, if we were provided sufficient resources. Paul B. Beeson, an American who was head physician in a Red Cross Harvard Field Hospital in England in World War II and later was the Nuffield Chair of Medicine at Oxford University, recognized this "can-do" spirit: "It was abundantly demonstrated during the war that if you put enough money into a big problem, you could solve it: radar, jet propulsion, penicillin" (Kaufman 1993).

The fourth theme is that serendipity plays a lead role in many scientific discoveries. Sometimes the same chance research findings have presented themselves to scientists from an earlier era, but their importance remains unappreciated until society (and scientists) are prepared to accept them. Louis Pasteur suggested that chance favors the prepared mind. Likewise, we also might conclude that chance favors the prepared society. Some discoveries must await changes in the scientists and the society before their practical application unfolds. In retelling the story of penicillin, we highlight these four themes, and we will refer to them frequently in Chapters 7 and 8 when discussing the discovery of drugs for mental illness.

The Story of Penicillin

In 1945, Alexander Fleming, Howard Florey, and Ernst Chain shared the Nobel Prize for the discovery of penicillin. Historians credit Fleming with discovering the antibacterial properties of *Penicillium* mold in 1928, even though other scientists had reported similar observations as much as 50 years earlier (Chain 1963; Weatherall 1990). By the late 1930s, René Dubos, working at the Rockefeller Institute, had concluded that since microorganisms eventually decompose all living substances, then soil must contain microorganisms that decompose bacteria (Weatherall 1990). Thus, early in the twentieth century, scientists already understood the idea of antibiosis. What scientists did not know was whether they could use these agents to kill bacteria without killing the patient.

There have been many entertaining accounts of how Fleming made his chance discovery of penicillin, although historians now suggest that many of these accounts were apocryphal (Macfarlane 1984; Le Fanu 1999). During the 1930s, scientists used the *Penicillium* mold to prevent the growth of contaminants in bacterial cultures. Howard Florey first collaborated with Fleming in work on the lysozyme properties of mucus while he was at Cambridge University (Macfarlane 1979). Florey subsequently moved to Oxford in 1935 where he recruited a biochemist, Ernst Chain, from Cambridge. In 1938, Florey and Chain at Oxford and Norman Heatley, a biochemist at Cambridge University, began to study *Penicillium* mold to "describe its antibiotic actions." The team did not set out with a purposeful agenda to synthesize a new medication to treat human infections, however (Macfarlane 1979).

The threat of an invasion or bombardment of Britain was real by this time. Florey, like Aubrey Lewis, sent his children to North America for safety. He and his team also discussed strategies for destroying their experimental results if the Nazis invaded. In May 1940, the team tested the efficacy of the penicillin preparation on mice infected with streptococcus. The results were compelling, and the team began contemplating clinical applications in humans. Florey, in particular, recognized the potential importance of penicillin in caring for war wounds and, therefore, its potential in the war effort (Richards 1964; Sheehan 1982; Williams 1984).

Although the researchers demonstrated the potential to treat infections in mice, there was no known process for producing penicillin in large quantities (Macfarlane 1979). In 1941, the investigators took their discovery to pharmaceutical companies in the United Kingdom and the United States and explained the volume of penicillin culture fluids that would be required to treat a serious human infection. Chain (1963) described the companies' reactions this way:

> This was an entirely impractical proposition, and, in fact, most pharmaceutical manufacturers at that time, in Britain as well as in the United States, though they showed polite interest in what was undoubtedly a very striking and most remarkable experimental result, considered the idea of developing the biological production process of penicillin to the stage where the substance could become a drug of practical value as completely unrealistic and Utopian.

Through a series of fortunate contacts that the Rockefeller Foundation had organized and financed, Florey and Heatley visited multiple industrial and governmental leaders in a whirlwind tour of the United States during the months before Pearl Harbor (Richards 1964). They eventually met with A. J. Moyer, an expert in deep-tank fermentation at the U.S. Department of Agriculture's North Regional Research Laboratory in Peoria, Illinois. Here the team identified a strain of *Penicillium* that produced even higher and more reproducible yields (Richards 1964). Perhaps most bizarre in the series of improbabilities at Peoria was that the researchers identified a culture medium that increased penicillin production by several orders of magnitude (Sheehan 1982). Peoria's North Regional Research Laboratory just happened to be charged with finding a commercial use for an extract that had been left over after producers extracted cornstarch from corn. This extract was piling up with no known use in the middle of one of the world's most productive corn belts.

The project was gathering momentum. The U.S. government created the Office of Scientific Research and Development to "initiate and support scientific research on medical problems affecting the national defense" (Sheehan 1982). This office provided and facilitated a forum that enabled several pharmaceutical companies to participate in an unprecedented cooperative venture. These companies took a big risk because, at the time, the scientific and pharmaceutical industries thought that researchers should focus resources on the chemical synthesis of penicillin, not on its microbial production (Sheehan 1982). The confluence of many other unique wartime anomalies were so important in this story that analysts have suggested that "penicillin is a direct result of the Second World War" (Chain 1963; Richards 1964; Williams 1984).

Commercially produced penicillin first became available in August 1942. A million units cost $200 in 1942 (about $1800 in 2001 dollars), and this was less than the price of production (Richards 1964). The price dropped to $35 by the following year ($285 in 1999 dollars) and to 50 cents by 1950 ($3.50 in 1999 dollars) (Richards 1964; Williams 1984). However, the limiting factor was availability, not cost. The federal government controlled the distribution of penicillin during World War II. By 1943, Paul Beeson had returned from the Red Cross Harvard Field hospital in England to accept a post as an infectious disease specialist at Emory University in Atlanta. One of Beeson's roles in this new post was to serve as the "drug czar of penicillin" for the entire southeastern portion of the United States. As Sheehan (1982) described:

The magic of [penicillin] endowed the people associated with it with glamour. Scientists studying penicillin became popular heroes; doctors who administered it became holy men; and, at least during the war years when penicillin was in desperately short supply, the man who controlled its distribution became a god.

Physicians from across the region called Beeson, requesting permission to use penicillin for a particular case and requesting access to the rationed stores of penicillin. Policy makers approved penicillin only for use in specific infections. The drug was both expensive and in low supply, so distributors denied many requests. Beeson recalled the following remarkable anecdote:

An episode I remember with clarity is that of a practitioner in another town calling me and saying he had a patient with syphilis and wanted to use penicillin for that, and I said, "No way, this drug is not to be used for syphilis because it has not been proved that it would be of any good." (Quoted in Kaufman 1993)

At this time, doctors still treated syphilis with drugs of the same class as those that Ehrlich had discovered 20 years earlier. Patients receiving these drugs required close monitoring, which led to the development of specialized syphilis clinics in most major cities. Neurosyphilis, a complication of syphilis, was a common reason for admission to the mental asylums in the first half of the twentieth century. In a few short years, penicillin would not only transform syphilis treatment, it also would help empty the asylums and transform the therapeutic and scientific approach to mental illness. We address that story in Chapter 7.

The success of penicillin stimulated a massive search for other antibiotics and medications, with a ripple effect continuing to this day. Streptomycin for tuberculosis, cortisone for inflammatory arthritis, vitamin B12, artificial kidneys, blood transfusions, and anesthesia all came of age during World War II. Perhaps even more remarkable is that each of these discoveries contained at least as many bizarre and mysterious episodes of happenstance, serendipity, and unexpected but seized opportunities as the discovery of penicillin. The story of penicillin is the prototype of academic-industry-government collaboration in the face of great necessity, the power of massive resources, and the role of serendipity.

The penicillin story also marked the transfer of leadership in biomedical research from the United Kingdom and Europe to the United States (Duffy 1993), which had been precipitated by the destruction of Europe's basic academic and industrial infrastructure and an influx of intellectual capital from Europe. Many stories of discovery have involved Jewish scientists forced by the Nazis from their homes, universities, and original fields of study. Other important factors contributing to the penicillin story included the U.S.'s growing financial capital, Americans' confidence in science, and the generosity of the government and philanthropy in supporting research (Weatherall 1990; Duffy 1993).

Backlash to the Therapeutic Revolution

These investments in biomedical research contributed to enormous health dividends. The average life expectancy in 1930 was about 60 years. By 1960 it increased to 70 years, and in 2001 it approached 80 years. Between 1920 and 1960, the death rate from tuberculosis fell from 113 per 100,000 to 6 per 100,000. The death rate from pneumonia/influenza and maternal complications during this period fell from 207 per 100,000 to 37 per 100,000 and from 70 per 100,000 to 37 per 100,000, respectively (Chain 1963). Infant mortality, deficiency states, malaria, and malnutrition also followed this pattern. The three leading causes of death in the first half of the twentieth century were all infectious diseases; by midcentury, these infectious diseases had been "conquered," and the three leading causes of death became heart disease, cancer, and stroke. Through a better understanding of how to prevent and treat infectious diseases, public health experts and medical science changed the major causes of death in industrialized societies. Instead of dying from infectious diseases such as tuberculosis at a young age, people began dying from chronic conditions such as heart disease at later ages.

This success ushered in new problems: an aging population, disabling chronic diseases, and increasing health-care costs. Given infectious diseases' enormous contribution to human suffering, industrialized nations expected that advances in their treatment would improve the human condition. This has undoubtedly happened, but not as a panacea. Commentators noted that "the decline in infectious diseases has not been accompanied, as many people had hoped, by a great reduction in the number of sick persons in the community, but by a change in the types of common disorders" (Wadsworth et al. 1971). Epidemiologists have described the rise in cardiovascular disease morbidity and mortality between the 1930s and 1960s, especially among older citizens, as an epidemic. This change in the epidemiology of disease led to two developments that have characterized the period from 1970 to the present. First, the "single acute disease, single infectious agent, and single magic bullet" framework gave way to a paradigm of complex, co-morbid, chronic diseases; multiple risk factors; and primary, secondary, and tertiary prevention strategies. Second, public opinion regarding the potential of big science and the aim of medicine grew more ambivalent. Both of these changes had an enormous influence on the day-to-day provision of primary health care.

The war on such problems as cardiovascular disease, cancer, muscular dystrophy, and dementia, for example, proved to be more intractable than the war on infectious diseases. Historians even scaled back the gains attributed to medical science for infectious diseases. Social scientists and others suggested that the massive improvement in mortality from infectious disease was due at least as much to improvements in hygiene and nutrition as it was from antibiotics (McKeown 1961; Le Fanu 1999). For example:

The marked improvement in health is attributable primarily, not to what happens when we are ill, but to the fact that we do not become ill. And the main reason why we do not become ill is because we live in a healthier environment. It is to environmental services and the favorable trend in the standard of living that we are largely indebted for our better health. Medical history, like common sense, suggests that in designing services we should seek to promote prevention of disease rather than its cure, domiciliary rather than institutional care and, within the hospital, a wide range of activities of which complex investigation and treatment of established disease are only a part. (McKeown 1961)

Drug therapies also suffered some crushing blows with the thalidomide disaster (a medication that caused deformed limbs in the children of women who took it early in pregnancy), psychotropic drug abuse (benzodiazepines, for example), and the perception of profit-making in the pharmaceutical industry. By the 1970s, an increasingly vocal group of academics and policy makers questioned the wisdom of public funding for health care and health-care research, and the physician's authoritative role came under scrutiny. Indeed, as Ann Cartwright's research demonstrated, patients began to question their physicians' decisions, judgments, and motives more closely (Cartwright and Anderson 1981).

Paul Beeson, who had been Chair of Medicine at both Yale and Oxford and the editor of several editions of *Cecil's Textbook of Medicine*, a leading medical textbook, attempted to provide some rational documentation of how medical care had improved. He compared the treatments suggested for common diseases in the first edition of the textbook in 1927 with the recommendations for treatment for these same diseases in 1975 (14th edition). He divided treatments into ten categories:

1. Recommended treatment now regarded as valueless
2. No effective treatment available
3. Treatment only marginally helpful at best
4. Measures available for relief of symptoms only
5. Treatment effective in limited circumstances
6. Prevention measures effective in limited circumstances
7. Treatment suppresses or controls the disease, but must be maintained long term
8. Ttreatment results in substantial improvements in the manifestations of the disease
9. Treatment is effective in most circumstances
10. Treatment is effective in prevention in most circumstances

Beeson found that treatments falling in categories 1–4 fell from 60% of the extant therapies in 1927 to 22% in 1975. Those in categories 5–6 fell from 34% to 28%. Categories 7–8 increased from 3% to 28%, and categories 9–10 increased from 3% to 22%. Beeson documented a decrease in the useless (or even harmful) therapies and a corresponding increase in effective therapies.

Beeson concluded that these were compelling data that demonstrated vast improvements in medical care. Indeed, the improvements are impressive from a historical perspective. From a twenty-first-century perspective, and especially from the perspective of a population dominated by persons born into a world where penicillin was commonplace and death from infectious diseases was not, these data give a "cup half-empty" impression. Nearly all the therapies in 1975 that rated the 9–10 status were either antimicrobial or vitamin treatments. In addition, with the enormous changes in medical education, regulatory oversight, and experimental methods, it is surprising to see that Beeson rated almost one-quarter of the available therapies for common diseases in 1975 as having no value or marginal value. In the 25 years since Beeson's report, scientists have replaced some of these marginal therapies with more effective interventions. However, policy makers increasingly have greeted newer therapies with suspicion.

Changing expectations also diminished the magnitude of these prior victories. Such problems as antibiotic resistance, the AIDS epidemic, flesh-eating bacteria, and mad cow disease shake our culture's perception of medicine's dominance over infectious diseases. Most physicians in practice today have not worked in a tuberculosis asylum, have not seen a child die of whooping cough, and have not seen even a single case of neurosyphilis. Preceptors must search the hospital to find enough patients with valvular heart disease to teach medical students the techniques of heart auscultation. The role of vaccines in decreasing childhood death is so underappreciated that some parents fail to take the simple step of having their children vaccinated against diphtheria, mumps, or polio. Young men in urban areas are more likely to die of gunshot wounds than from influenza, and young women are more likely to die in a motor vehicle accident than in childbirth. Most physicians have never attended a death in a home. Successful aging, preventive health, exercise, and nutrition have become part of the popular culture.

Chronic disease replaced acute disease as people's most common reason to visit a primary-care physician. It is difficult to overestimate the importance of this change on the daily practice of medicine. Efforts to improve the care of patients with chronic disease push generalist physicians into disease prevention, and this compels them to become more involved in multiple determinants of health. This new responsibility demands that physicians play a larger role in their patients' lifestyle decisions. The story of cardiovascular disease best exemplifies physicians' increasing role the lives of people and their communities. The path of discovery and changes in public policy for cardiovascular disease parallels the one that science and society will retrace for depression.

The Story of Cardiovascular Disease

Evidence about chronic disease prevention began pointing scientists to interventions aimed at lifestyle behaviors, such as smoking, diet, and physical activity. Although there was a public backlash against the physician's authoritative role, the cost of medical care, and the cost of research, the new banner of prevention took some of the bite out of these criticisms. Prevention resulted not only in funding some of the largest and most expensive clinical trials of all time (Le Fanu 1999), it also led to an intrusion of providers into asymptomatic individuals' daily lives. Providers increasingly made patients responsible for self-care and for strict adherence to long-term intervention strategies. The story of cardiovascular disease exemplifies the new prevention approach.

Soon after the end of World War II, an alarming statistic came to the public's attention: Half of all deaths were due to cardiovascular disease. In 1947, the United States established the National Heart Institute to organize and fund the war on heart disease. The first major project of this Institute was the Framingham Study. Many view this study as giving rise to the notion of risk factors and as initiating the systematic study of the causes of common chronic diseases. However, some authorities point to epidemiological studies championed by the U.S. health insurance industry as the true beginning of this movement. The first large-scale studies of blood pressure have been attributed to insurance companies, culminating with a 1939 publication that presented pooled data from 15 companies representing 1.3 million subjects. These data showed an unequivocal association between high blood pressure and early mortality (Lew 1973; Postel-Vinay 1996).

Early debates about hypertension paralleled those about depression. For example, is an elevated blood pressure due more to social, environmental, or biological causes? There was also considerable discussion about whether physicians could best treat hypertension with psychological as opposed to medical therapies:

Critical review of the available evidence suggests that hypertension is a disease peculiarly responsive to social and emotional influences, although the relationships of these to the genetic substrate, to early interpersonal experiences, to the formation of predisposing unconscious conflicts, and to the precipitation and maintenance of the hypertensive state are largely unknown. (Woods et al. 1958)

Scientists specifically designed the Framingham study to identify the differences between individuals who developed cardiovascular disease and those who did not. Over the next 30 years, this study contributed information on the risk factors for heart disease and innovations in designing research studies. This included new statistical methods for modeling risk, interactive and multifactorial risk profiles, health screening, prediction of future risk, and the potential for prevention at an early, asymptomatic stage of illness (Dawber 1980; Kannel 1992; Kannel and Larson 1993). In the past decade, ideas about early prevention have even come to include the potential for preventing adult diseases through changes in embryonic and fetal development (Barker and Osmond 1992).

The Framingham Study, among multiple others, established high serum cholesterol, hypertension, diabetes, cigarette smoking, and family history as the major risk factors for cardiovascular disease. Scientists already had linked smoking to the epidemic of lung cancer and chronic obstructive pulmonary disease, though they had not produced research on how to help people stop smoking. Scientists had linked diabetes with kidney disease, but the idea that tight control of blood sugar might prevent end-organ damage was unproved. When researchers discovered thiazide diuretics (while searching for a treatment for a different problem), hypertension became a logical target for intervention and, in turn, stimulated further research on other drugs for high blood pressure. When researchers suggested that diet alone did not correct high-serum cholesterol, they began researching cholesterol-lowering agents. Researchers required a huge amount of funding to test the efficacy of the new medications that they hoped would modify these risk factors. In turn, public policy makers translated these findings into major public health campaigns against smoking in the 1960s, hypertension in the 1970s, and cholesterol in the 1980s.

Scientists next discovered how risk factors interact with genetic and environmental factors. They then moved from studies that each addressed a single risk factor to studies addressing multiple risk factors. At the time, the Multiple Risk Factor Intervention Trial (MRFIT) in the United States was the most expensive clinical trial ever conducted (Le Fanu 1999). In the United Kingdom, Geoffrey Rose was leading the World Health Organization–sponsored European Collaborative Trial in the Multifactorial Prevention of Coronary Heart Disease. In the 1950s and 1960s, Rose, a neuropsychiatrist in the Royal Air Force in World War II and a trainee of George Pickering at Oxford, had conducted epidemiological studies of hypertension. These multiple-risk-factor trials demonstrated that subjects who were able to reduce their risk profiles did indeed decrease their risk of cardiovascular mortality (Kornitzer 1992). These studies also supported two of Rose's (1992) principles regarding screening and treating diseases. First, screening for multifactorial diseases should be multifactorial. In the case of cardiovascular disease, it does not make sense to screen for cholesterol but not smoking. A patient's risk results from all the relevant factors: "Our aim should be to identify risk, not the individual risk factor." Second, prevention of a multifactorial disease must be multifactorial. It makes little sense to concentrate on lipids and ignore smoking, diabetes, and hypertension. We will argue later in this book that the current treatment model for emotional disorders fails to incorporate these lessons.

By the 1970s, epidemiologists described coronary heart disease as a worldwide epidemic. Rose went on to play a leadership role in the World Health Organization's global efforts to prevent heart disease. The notion of a global community and a global burden of disease began through efforts to eradicate malaria, yellow fever, and other infectious diseases. After the World Health Organization succeeded in infectious disease control, cardiovascular disease became one of its next targets. Its ability to conduct cross-cultural studies provided the framework for collecting evidence on the variation in rates of disease and the prevalence of risk factors. These types of studies provided a template for future cross-cultural studies investigating risk factors for cancer, neurological disease, schizophrenia, and eventually depression.

Scientists next moved from studies targeting patients at high risk for cardiovascular disease to studies of risk reduction for the larger group of patients who had only moderate or low risk. Concomitantly, experts suggested a progressive lowering of the acceptable ranges of serum glucose, serum cholesterol, and blood pressure values. George Pickering had suggested at mid-century that blood pressure was normally distributed across the population, challenging the notion of a bimodal distribution of blood pressure and the idea of a critical value indicating disease (Oldham 1960). Rose (1985) took this hypothesis a step further by introducing the notion of a "sick population." This hypothesis stemmed from observations of the Framingham cohort, among others. Even though investigators could identify a "low-risk" group of patients compared to those with high risk for coronary artery disease, the leading cause of death in the low-risk group was still coronary artery disease. In other words, if you are a 60-year-old Anglo-American with no cardiac risk factors, you are still most likely to die of cardiovascular disease. Rose and others raised concern over the false sense of security evoked when a doctor tells a patient that his or her "cholesterol is normal." Rose thus introduced the notion of "mass strategy," which suggests that a large group of people with a small risk of disease generates more cases of disease than a small group of people at the highest risk.

Mass Strategy

Mass strategy emanates from the principle that having many subjects exposed to a small risk generates more cases of disease than having a few subjects exposed to a high risk (Rose 1992). This concept is relevant to the issue of severe psychiatric disease compared to mild to moderate psychiatric illness. Unfortunately for prevention efforts, using a mass strategy leads to the prevention paradox, which suggests that "a preventive measure which brings much benefit to the population offers little benefit to each individual" (Rose 1992). Conversely, a strategy of prevention that targets high-risk individuals offers definite rewards to those individuals, but is only weakly effective at reducing the societal burden of disease. Thus, in the latest chapter of the prevention story, physicians like Rose assume an activist role in changing the lifestyles of communities. At this point, the clinician and the scientist move into the murky and mercurial waters of the cultural and political maelstrom, often as the uninvited bearers of bad news and with little practical experience. Medical intervention at the community level raises important issues about the aims of medicine:

This population approach to prevention takes us beyond the responsibilities of medicine. The underlying causes for the rise and fall of major diseases, and for their national and regional differences, are related to the circumstances and manner of daily life. It is the responsibility of doctors to communicate their findings and expert opinions to the public and their governments, to exhort and support, and (if possible) to set a good personal example of healthy life-style, but society, not doctors, must decide how it wishes to live and what its priorities are. The prevention of heart disease is basically a matter of social, economic, and political policy. (Rose 1992)

The story of cardiovascular disease stands as a model for a huge number of subsequent epidemiological studies investigating risk factors for diseases, ranging from cancer to birth defects to peptic ulcers to depression. It also serves as a model for identifying and promoting protective factors and healthy lifestyles throughout a population. Physical activity and meditation for heart disease are similar to antioxidants, clean water, and fiber for cancer prevention, along with a spectrum of other protective strategies ranging from seat belts to natural foods. In areas where these recommendations conflict with cultural norms and personal desires, medicine must ponder the boundaries of patient advocacy. Although we outline the cardiovascular disease story as if it were a logical progression of science and fact, considerable controversy still exists about its causes and treatments.

Many of these controversies have analogs in the story of depression, and we therefore highlight them briefly here. Many patients at risk for heart disease have no symptoms. In fact, the medicines they may take to prevent heart disease actually may give them undesirable symptoms. People without symptoms are thereby taught that they are sick. Furthermore, we may teach these people that their lifestyle behaviors and personal choices are responsible for their illness. Taken to an extreme, patients can be blamed for their illnesses. Aronowitz (1998) noted the powerful influence of social norms on views about diagnosing and treating cardiovascular disease. This etiology of personal responsibility tends to underemphasize the role of societal and environmental factors. In the case of hypertension, for example, is the stress of poverty the "cause" of the illness, or is the cause the individual's high-salt diet? Does labeling the problem as a lifestyle choice medicalize what is actually a social problem? If the cause of the hypertension is the stress of poverty, is this the purview of generalist physicians?

People worry that too much power has been placed in the hands of scientists and physicians (Le Fanu 1999). This power gives scientists and physicians too much authority to make decisions about who is sick and how they should be labeled and treated. This power also enables scientists to decide what types of research for new treatments are socially acceptable (for example, stem cell research). Concentrating social influence in the hand of scientists and physicians draws particular concern and scorn when it is coupled with the perception of conflicts of interest. These conflicts of interest appear in two major forms. First, there is a concern that the pharmaceutical industry unduly influences physicians' decisions about who is sick and how they should be treated. Second, there is a concern that decisions about how resources are distributed are influenced by special interest groups rather that the frequency or severity of particular diseases. All these issues have analogs in the controversies that surround the treatment of emotional disorders.

Summary

By the 1980s, mass strategies, disease management, and health-promotion strategies resulted in at least five changes in the primary-care delivery system.

1. Primary-care physicians took responsibility for the long-term management of a large group of patients with asymptomatic conditions that are harbingers of serious illness. Part of this role involved educating and cajoling patients to assume difficult lifestyle changes in order to realize uncertain future gains.
2. Primary-care physicians conducted a large-scale screening operation for asymptomatic conditions and risky behaviors.
3. Primary-care physicians took responsibility for the long-term management of symptomatic and disabling chronic conditions.
4. Primary-care physicians took responsibility for the use of many new diagnostic and screening tests to accomplish their new responsibilities.
5. Society expanded the primary-care physician–patient dyad to include the health-care team and external regulators.

Using a mass strategy places the primary-care physician in a sometimes unfamiliar and sometimes unwelcome role of social activist. In this chapter we provided a glimpse into fundamental changes in the practice of primary-care medicine. This began with discoveries in public health measures and medical therapeutics and resulted in a dramatic change in the leading causes of morbidity and mortality. When psychiatry brings its new innovations to primary care, it does so in the context of these dramatic changes. We now turn the fundamental changes in the practice of psychiatry and the treatment of severe mental illness.

7

THE FALL AND RISE OF SPECIALTY PSYCHIATRY

The goal of this chapter is not to give a detailed history of psychiatry or psychopharmacology. Those histories are well recorded. Rather, we briefly review the developments in psychiatry over the past half-century as they pertain to reinventing depression in primary care, societal views of psychiatry and mental illness, and psychiatry's shift in focus from severe mental illness in asylums to milder forms in primary care. We also describe the development of the first effective drugs for mental illness, both to draw parallels with the discoveries outlined in the previous chapter and to show how these drugs emboldened psychiatry to expand its reach into primary care.

A Critique of Psychiatry

In the 1940s, most people viewed mental illness as irreversible; it carried enormous social stigma and the morbid dread of potential institutionalization. The ideas that mental illness could derange part of the mind and not other parts, and that treatment could remedy the deranged part, were new at mid-century. Although the view that an individual could have a disorder of emotion while the rest of his mind remained intact had been established during the first half of the nineteenth century (Berrios 2000), the "all-or-none" view of madness remained inscribed in popular culture into the twentieth century.

Society misunderstood and mistrusted psychiatry in general and the psychoanalytic approach in particular. Joseph Heller was a bombardier in World War II. Although his novel *Catch-22* (1962) stands as a metaphor for the distrust of power that epitomized the 1960s, his caricatures of authority, physicians, and psychiatry arose from his 1940s wartime experience. In the scene retold below, Yossarian, the bombardier, has been discussing his concern about the wisdom of allowing his pilot (Orr) to continue to fly. He has voiced this concern to Doc Daneeka, the physician at the military air base in Europe. Doc Daneeka is a pathetic physician who spends all of his time worrying about himself and his income. Doc Daneeka has just finished explaining why he will allow Orr to continue to pilot Yossarian's plane. Yossarian recapitulates the explanation as follows:

There was only one catch and that was Catch-22, which specified that a concern for one's own safety in the face of dangers that were real and immediate was the process of a rational mind. Orr was crazy and could be grounded. All he had to do was ask; and as soon as he did, he would no longer be crazy and would have to fly more missions. Orr would be crazy to fly more missions and sane if he didn't, but if he was sane he had to fly them. If he flew them he was crazy and didn't have to. Yossarian was moved very deeply by the absolute simplicity of this clause of Catch-22 and let out a respectful whistle.

The view of mental illness portrayed in this passage demonstrates society's ambivalence toward psychiatry as a science. Psychiatry had two fundamental tasks at mid-century. One was to change centuries-old public and professional opinions regarding the prevalence, etiology, and reversibility of psychiatric illness. The second was to demonstrate that psychiatric theory and treatments emanated from the same scientific origins and evidence as treatments for medical illness. Psychiatric researchers had to take therapies out of the black box and communicate to the broader professional and lay audiences, using standard biomedical principles. Put another way, in the early 1940s, psychiatry was outside mainstream medicine, and other providers viewed psychiatrists as the administrators of warehouses of mental illness, which were viewed as asylums at best and snake pits at worst (Gorman 1956). People viewed mental illness as "irreversible," which arose from historical and quasi-religious notions about the indivisibility of the soul. Some of these generalizations stemmed from repeated personal observations of people rarely recovering from psychiatric illness and rarely leaving the asylums.

At the 100th anniversary of the American Psychiatric Association in 1944, Alan Gregg, Director for Medical Sciences at the Rockefeller Foundation in New York, delivered a critique of psychiatry:

No other specialty of medicine has had a history so strange, nor a relation to human thought so intimate, as psychiatry. The three most powerful traditions or historical heritages of psychiatry are still, as they have been from time immemorial, the horror which mental disease inspires, the power and subtlety with which psychiatric symptoms influence human relations, and the tendency of man to think of spirit as not only separable from but already separate from body. These are the inherent, the inveterate, the inevitable handicaps of psychiatry.

In reviewing these heritages of psychiatry, the horror of psychiatric disease, the subtle confusion of early pathological signs with moral weakness or unethical behavior, and the false distinctions between mind and body, let me observe that no other specialty of medicine has had to rescue its patients from persecution, live with them in social ostracism, restore their capacities and then return them to an environment both exigent and suspicious. If we realize that man is always superstitious and irrationally conservative when he is beset by fear and crisis, then it is a wonder that scientific medicine has ever emerged from witchcraft. And it is yet more remarkable that diseases producing mental and spiritual signs and symptoms have ever been dealt with rationally and scientifically.

Asylums at this time cared not only for patients with schizophrenia but also for sizable populations of patients with neurological damage from trauma, syphilis, meningitis, alcohol, senile dementia, and other neurological illnesses. The approach to treatment, which was largely supportive, was similar across these diseases that we now recognize as very dissimilar. Neither the public nor the profession appeared interested or capable of distinguishing among the major categories of psychiatric or neurological illness. Doctors viewed psychoses, seizures, and focal neurological deficits due to neurosyphilis ("general paresis of the insane") in the same light as psychoses due to schizophrenia, seizures due to head trauma, and paresis due to meningitis. Because there were no specific treatments, providers found specific diagnoses irrelevant.

Society believed that people inherited psychiatric illness and that it was irreversible. The remnants of "degeneration theory" suggested to many that any psychiatric illness in the family would become worse with each successive generation. For these reasons, not only did patients fear a diagnosis of insanity and the stigma of institutionalization, but also their families were at risk. Who would want to marry the sister of a young man in an asylum, knowing that her children were doomed to the same fate?

Asylum psychiatry provided custodial care, and doctors offered treatment with barbiturates and bromides. They protected the patient while everyone waited, hoped, and prayed for a spontaneous recovery. Asylums were an important improvement in the care of such patients, compared with their persecution, imprisonment, or neglect in earlier eras. Still, there were ample examples of abuse, negligence, unethical incarceration, overcrowding, and inhumane conditions to frighten both patients and professionals. By the beginning of World War II, most in psychiatry understood that asylum psychiatry had failed:

In the first half of the twentieth century, psychiatry was caught in a dilemma. On the one hand, psychiatrists could warehouse their patients in vast bins in the hopes that they might recover spontaneously. On the other, they had psychoanalysis, a therapy suitable for the needs of wealthy people desiring self-insight, but not for real psychiatric illness. Caught between these unappealing choices, psychiatrists sought alternatives. Some of these alternatives proved to be dead ends and were discarded; others became the basis of a new vision of psychotherapy; still others laid the groundwork for the revolution in drug therapy that would take place after World War II. (Shorter 1997)

The best measure of the sense of futility that psychiatrists experienced in caring for these patients was the shear number (and often the incredible toxicity) of attempted treatments. These were desperate measures for dreaded conditions, and scientists foisted hundreds of different treatments on thousands of patients over several decades. This was a trial-and-error exercise on a massive scale. Hydrotherapy, laxatives, purgatives, iatrogenic abscesses, partial colectomy, caffeine, opium, sedatives, bromides, prolonged narcosis, lobotomy, and various forms of shock therapy comprise a short list of approaches that enjoyed brief popularity. Physicians still used prolonged narcosis, or sleep therapy (in which, using sedative drugs or narcotics, the patient was induced into a long period of sleep which was believed to be therapeutic), until World War II, although researchers progressively improved the safety of agents used to induce sleep. Psychotherapy was controversial, not only because of criticisms arising from analysts external to the movement but also due to arguments among the various camps promoting different forms of psychotherapy. In his critique of psychiatry, Gregg (1944) summed up psychiatrists' problems in this manner:

My own formulation of your major limitations would be this: you are badly recruited, you are isolated from medicine, you are overburdened, and you are too inarticulate and long-suffering to secure redress from the public of some of the handicaps from which you and your patients suffer.

Why is it news to so many citizens in this over-informed and unreflecting country that we use more hospital beds for your specialty than for all the rest of medicine . . . all put together?

Psychiatrists did not brush off Gregg's criticisms because he had been a long time supporter of psychiatric research through funding from the Rockefeller Foundation. At the same time, he was not beholden to any particular psychiatric dogma, school of thought, or academic unit. The committee responsible for his invitation to speak requested Gregg's frank critique because they viewed him as being at once an insider and an outsider. By the end of the war, many more Americans understood the magnitude of the suffering and costs associated with psychiatric illness, as well as the need for improved treatments.

The Dawn of Physical Treatments

The first effective physical treatment in psychiatry originated in the late nineteenth century, when a Viennese psychiatrist, Julius Wagner-Jauregg, noted that one of his psychotic patients achieved a remission when she contracted erysipelas in 1883 (Stone 1997; Shorter 1997). As there were already extant theories about a relationship between fever and psychosis, he hypothesized that the heat-sensitive syphilis spirochete might be amenable to treatment by inducing fever. Recall that Ehrlich's Salvarsan had already been available for several years, but it was most useful in preventing neurosyphilis. Thus, neurosyphilis was a desperate disease with essentially 100% mortality. Wagner-Jauregg initially attempted to induce fever among patients with neurosyphilis using the tuberculin vaccine, but it was too toxic. In 1917, he injected the blood of a patient with malaria into patients with neurosyphilis, and they improved. Wagner-Jauregg won the Nobel Prize for this work 10 years later. "Fever cure" was the first specific remedy for a specific psychiatric illness. Physicians administered "fever cure" to other patients with myriad psychiatric illnesses, but it proved effective only for neurosyphilis. Twenty-five years later, in Atlanta, Paul Beeson was still using fever cure as the standard treatment for patients with neurosyphilis. By this time, the less toxic typhoid vaccine was the agent used to induce the fever, but the concept was the same. Even after penicillin and antipsychotics were discovered, fever cure was still under investigation in the 1960s (Lehmann 1960).

The story of convulsive therapy followed the same path as the new treatment discovery outlined in the previous chapter. Scientists discovered insulin in 1922, and in the late 1920s, Manfred Sakel, an Austrian psychiatrist, began using insulin to help manage the symptoms of morphine withdrawal (Shorter 1997). Why he thought it might be useful is unclear. Some patients inadvertently developed insulin coma during this treatment. Curiously, Sakel noted that patients enjoyed tranquillity when they came out of the coma. He then hypothesized that this tranquillity might be therapeutic for the agitation of schizophrenia. Sakel subsequently reported that the treatment was effective, but reviewers denounced his results, while the therapy diffused slowly and only in isolated pockets throughout the world.

In a parallel development, a neuropathologist in Budapest, Ladislas von Meduna, reported that brain specimens of patients who had suffered from epilepsy differed from those of patients who had suffered from schizophrenia. He hypothesized that seizures might antagonize the process of schizophrenia. In 1934, he began inducing seizures with medications as a treatment for schizophrenia. Then in the following year, a team of Italian scientists began using electricity to induce experimental seizures in animals in an effort to understand the pathophysiology of epilepsy. Through a series of hunches and with the knowledge of the effectiveness of convulsive therapies, they hypothesized that this might help treat schizophrenia.

In 1938, the team reported the results of electroshock, or electroconvulsive therapy (ECT) (Berrios 1997). With pre-treatment muscle relaxants, ECT became the shock treatment of choice by the 1950s, as opposed to the convulsions induced by medications or the shock induced by insulin (Shorter 1997; Stone 1997). As we now know, however, ECT is not effective for treating schizophrenia. In the early 1940s, Lothar B. Kalinowsky, yet another scientist fleeing the Nazis, conducted clinical evaluations of ECTs in the United States, parallel to those of L. H. Smith in the United Kingdom. These studies demonstrated that ECT was effective only for major depression (Robinson 1978; Berrios 1997).

At the beginning of World War II, the treatments available to psychiatrists included psychoanalysis and other forms of psychotherapy; prolonged narcosis; insulin shock; abreactive techniques; social services interventions; and various forms of recreational, occupational, and physical therapy (Bartemeier et al. 1946). ECT became more accepted, and physicians could apply fever cure for neurosyphilis. Except for the psychiatrists who practiced outpatient psychoanalysis, psychiatrists conducted most psychiatric practice in asylum settings for the severely mentally ill. Neurologists, pathologists, and neuroanatomists led most of the research on psychiatric illness.

By the end of World War II, psychiatry had completed a fundamental reformation on three fronts. First, it promoted an improved professional and public understanding of the prevalence, causes, morbidity, and treatability of psychiatric illness. Second, it won greater sympathy and understanding for patients with psychiatric illness. Third, society found greater appreciation for the field of psychiatry. Much of this reformation had its roots in the flood of psychiatric casualties in World War II.

The Stress of War on Soldiers

Psychiatrist and military leaders recognized the magnitude of psychological stress under battlefield conditions during the World War I. These casualties fell within the framework of "shell shock" in contrast to the "combat fatigue" of soldiers in World War II. Experts viewed shell shock as a direct effect of bombshell explosions. These explosions caused an immediate effect on the central nervous system in a susceptible host. Writing in 1919, H. C. Marr describes the distinction as follows:

Simple neurasthenia is a weakness of the neurons of the cerebrospinal axis. In its mental aspects it is characterized by mild depression, lethargy, apathy, and retardation of memory. Simple neurasthenia arises as a result of mental stress and strain and physical ailments of manifold variety, acting particularly on persons with an inherited neurotic and neuropathic tendency. The weakness of the central nervous system lowers the tone of the body generally, primarily in the regions subserved by the sympathetic nervous system; it opens the way to the passage of organisms or poisonous products into the circulation, and induces the phenomenon of toxic neurasthenia. In the majority of the cases of so called shell shock, the effect of the explosion of the shell brings on the condition of toxic neurasthenia more suddenly; it accelerates the evolution of neurasthenia from the simple to the toxic form.

Physicians believed that the force of the explosion (or the physical trauma to soldiers temporarily buried alive under dirt and debris) exerted direct effects on the autonomic nervous system. During World War I there were more casualties due to tuberculosis and shell shock than to physical injuries. Psychiatrists prepared a report to the armed forces to help them better prepare for future psychiatric casualties. Unfortunately, these recommendations sat on the shelf for the early part of World War II (Ridenour 1961).

In World War II, shell shock was replaced with "combat fatigue" and in the Royal Air Force by the damning category of "low moral fiber." Doctors viewed the condition as caused by the cumulative effect of severe stress rather than the proximate physical result of the shelling. Indeed, the condition often appeared when combatants returned to the field after leave or during periods of stalemate when combat always seemed imminent. In contrast to the etiology that Marr posited, military psychiatrists in World War II explained that "the key to an understanding of the psychiatric problem is the simple fact that the danger of being killed or maimed imposes a strain so great that it causes men to break down. Psychiatric casualties are as inevitable as gunshot and shrapnel wounds in warfare" (Appel and Beebe 1946). These psychiatrists reported that a soldier's response was dose dependent and that everyone had a breaking point, regardless of their intrinsic and extrinsic defenses:

Practically all men in rifle battalions who were not otherwise disabled ultimately became psychiatric casualties. The average point at which this occurred appears to have been in the region of 200 to 240 aggregate combat days. Most of the men were ineffective [combatants] after 180 days. (Appel and Beebe 1946)

Doctors at the front lines used the term "combat fatigue" or "combat exhaustion" as an expedient label (Bartemeier et al. 1946). They chose these words over terms like "neurosis" or "anxiety" to avoid the possible labeling of men who returned to the combat areas. Military psychiatrists saw those men who required further evaluation and treatment, and they diagnosed these cases with traditional psychiatric labels. Notably, the overwhelming majority of these diagnoses consisted of mild to moderate cases of neurasthenia, anxiety, and personality disorders, rather than the civilian psychiatrist's typical regimen of psychoses. This exposed a large cadre of military psychiatrists to the much more common range of mild to moderate emotional disorders. Indeed, many of the affected men saw their symptoms resolve when they were removed from the source of the stress, plus had some sleep, a decent meal, and some kind words.

The stress of war, however, is only part of the story. Of all American men screened for enlistment between January 1942 and December 1945, the military rejected 1,875,000 because of neuropsychiatric disorders (Menninger 1947b). This represented 12% of all men examined and 37% of all men rejected for service. The military discharged another 517,000 from active duty due to neuropsychiatric illness; 39% of all medical discharges were for neuropsychiatric disorders. These figures do not include those men who rested for several days and then returned to the battle, nor do they include men who would have been psychiatric cases had they not been killed first. The British and Canadian Armed Forces reported figures of similar magnitude (Menninger 1947b).

The total number of men diagnosed with combat fatigue is unknown. Treatment for these casualties included rest, hot food, reassurance, and a facilitated return to combat. Psychiatrists sent those who did not improve with conservative measures to military hospitals. Doctors admitted one million men to hospitals during the war for treatment of neuropsychiatric illness. The military broadcast these figures and findings on the home front, but the public responded to these numbers by keeping in mind that those affected were their fathers, brothers, and husbands rather than an anonymous group of lunatics in distant asylums. Also, the notion that these illnesses were induced as a result of "fatigue" inflicted by fighting for one's country also helped reduce the stigma of mental illness.

Psychiatrists' ability to efficiently screen for psychiatric illness before enlistment was a major success for psychiatry in World War II. Among enlisted soldiers, military planners used preventive measures adopted at the suggestion of military psychiatrists to reduce the number of men suffering combat fatigue. These measures included reducing the number of days of exposure to combat, early treatment at facilities near the combat zones, and educating officers on strategies to improve morale (Appel and Beebe 1946). These prevention techniques proved to be successful, both in reducing the incidence of combat fatigue and in rehabilitating the soldiers so they could return to active duty. In other words, those with combat fatigue were often recognized and treated before the condition had reached a severe stage. The primary care and psychiatry literature seems to have forgotten this important story of successful preventive psychiatry.

Military doctors returned more than 80% of men with combat fatigue to active duty, and psychiatry enjoyed the accolades of the military leadership for these efforts (Bartemeier et al. 1946). World War II not only revealed the large number of people in the community at risk for mental illness, it also provided the field of psychiatry with credibility in identifying and caring for these people.

This returns us to the penicillin story discussed earlier. By the middle of 1943, the Office of Scientific Research and Development secured enough penicillin to organize a multi-site clinical trial of the antibiotic's effectiveness for a broad range of infections (Richards 1964). By the middle of 1944, scientists established penicillin as an effective treatment for syphilis. Even patients with neurosyphilis experienced improvement. This was the first example of a specific "magic bullet" for a psychiatric illness: "These were stunning stories. Neurosyphilis had once filled the asylums. Here was a definitive demonstration that one cause of insanity, at least, was curable" (Shorter 1997). The discovery of penicillin was the beginning of the end of the age of asylums and the beginning of specific therapies for specific psychiatric illnesses.

Backlash to the Expansion of Psychiatry

Psychiatry, or specifically, asylum psychiatry, had been under siege for some time, but World War II had another unintended effect. During this war, men who were conscientious objectors served as orderlies in the asylums, and this represented an important influx of observers into a system not normally visited or viewed by otherwise healthy young men. Several of these orderlies became articulate and forceful commentators about the deplorable asylum conditions. The bad publicity, coupled with increasing costs and new medications, led to the decline of asylums and the rise of community psychiatry in the 1950s and 1960s. As enlightened as this movement seemed at the time, its failure now stands as one of the black marks on the history of psychiatry. Historians suggest that this failure was as much the government's failure as it was psychiatrists'. In both the United States and the United Kingdom, psychiatrists discharged large numbers of patients from the asylums, but there was no infrastructure to provide for their mental health care in the community (Sedgewick 1982; Scull 1989; Grob 1994). Thus, an important success story turned into a debacle that helped fuel the antipsychiatry movement.

Psychiatry's role during World War II also initiated criticism of the profession. Was psychiatry merely acting as an agent of the military leadership in patching up men who were ill and vulnerable and returning them to the battlefield where many of them died? Did psychiatrists treat these men as military machinery no different from tanks and jeeps? Did psychiatry send these men back to combat too soon, when their psychiatric illness made them more susceptible to injury and death? With the end of the war, the advent of psychopharmacology, and the economy's conversion to peacetime expansion, critics reformulated this same argument as follows:

The concept of man as a robot was both an expression of and a powerful motive force in industrialized mass society. It was the basis for behavioral engineering in commercial, economic, political, and other advertising and propaganda; the expanding economy of the "affluent society" could not subsist without such manipulation. Only by manipulating humans ever more into Skinnerian rats, robots, buying automata, homeostatically adjusted conformers and opportunists (or, blunting speaking, into morons and zombies) can this great society follow its progress toward ever increasing gross national product. As a matter of fact, the principles of academic psychology were identical with those of the "pecuniary conception of man." (Bertalanffy 1968)

The achievements of psychiatry during World War II emboldened the profession to broaden its influence. Speaking at the Annual Meeting of the American Psychiatry Association soon after the war, William C. Menniger, who had been the highest-ranking psychiatrist in the U.S. Armed Forces, laid out a bold postwar challenge to his colleagues:

To some of us psychiatry seems to be at a crossroads: we may continue to permit our chief emphasis of interest to be in the psychoses or in seeing 6 to 8 analytic patients a day in our ivory towers. We can go on talking our jargon and accepting the trickle of all comers for our ranks. On the other hand we can turn up the road which leads us into the broad field of social interests: we can devote our efforts to the potential opportunities of helping the average man on the street. . . . We are living in a world filled with the residual of grief and sorrow and suffering that have nothing to do with "dementia praecox" or the "Oedipus conflict" but with individual struggles, community needs, state and national problems, and international concerns. (Bartemeier et al. 1946)

John Rawlings Rees, the leader of psychiatric services for the British Military, also encouraged an expanded role for psychiatry in curing societal problems in his 1945 book, *The Shaping of Psychiatry by War*. In his review of the book in the *British Medical Journal*, S. M. Coleman congratulated psychiatry for its wartime success but also chastised the author for overstretching the boundaries of his profession: "a shoemaker should stick to his last." In other words, psychiatry should maintain its focus on severe mental illness.

The criticisms about the direction and tools of psychiatry were as caustic from the inside as the outside. In his autobiography, William Sargant described a philosophical rift soon after World War II between the members of his group, which favored physical methods of treatment, and their former colleagues in the Maudsley Hospital. Sargant, the co-author of several editions of *An Introduction to Physical Methods of Treatment in Psychiatry* (Sargant and Slater 1954), wrote:

Many psychiatrists felt outraged to see its delicate and metaphysical host, the mind, ruthlessly handled by people who dared to suggest that psychiatry should be as direct in its approach as general medicine, and that the mind (conceived merely as the brain) would in the end be treated as practically as the liver, the lungs, and all similar organs.

Aubrey Lewis (at the Maudsley Hospital) (1945) remarked that the use of physical treatments was "untainted by the normal requirements of rational scientific skepticism." Notably, Sargant had been an early proponent of not only insulin shock and related therapies, but also ECT and leucotomy (a form of brain surgery). He also described his difficulties in winning approval from hospital officials to provide these treatments, while patients' families begged him for these interventions. The postwar period was rife with intraprofessional rivalries and debates regarding the role of psychotherapy versus psychoanalysis versus physical treatments. Psychopharmacology, however, would soon overshadow all three of these schools of thought. We turn now to the history of the accession of psychopharmacology in psychiatry.

The Genesis of Antidepressant Pharmacotherapy

There are at least three different accounts of the genesis of antidepressant pharmacotherapy. All three accounts fit within the archetypal model of discovery described in the story of penicillin. The first story is that of an Australian physician and former Japanese prisoner of war who began injecting schizophrenic patients' urine into the abdomens of guinea pigs, hoping to identify the toxic substance that causes schizophrenia. Instead, he stumbled onto a treatment for mania. The second story began with a pharmaceutical company experimenting on potential uses for excess Nazi rocket fuel in its search of a new treatment for tuberculosis. During human testing, it found that some of these substances induce euphoria in patients with tuberculosis, and thus the company decided to use the drug for depression. The third story involved a French military surgeon who was exploring the use of an antihistamine to prevent cardiovascular shock among anesthetized war casualties. In clinical tests, he noted that the drug produced "uninterest" in patients who were undergoing surgery, and then the drug was tested in patients with psychosis. These stories mark the humble beginnings of lithium, monoamine oxidase inhibitors, and chlorpromazine, respectively.

The Story of Lithium

In World War II, John F. Cade, a physician in the Australian military, was a prisoner of war for three-and-a-half years. During his time as a prisoner of war, he noted that many of the prisoners who suffered from functional psychoses also suffered from medical illnesses. He hypothesized that "mania might represent a state of intoxication arising as a result of an excess of some normal metabolite, whilst depression represented the effect of abnormally low levels of the same metabolite" (Johnson 1984). Cade returned to Melbourne after his release determined to explore this hypothesis. He was not at an academic institution and had no access to a true laboratory. He described his laboratory as "a bench, sink, a few jars of chemicals, some simple lab instruments (pipettes, etc.) and the guinea pigs. These were housed in our back garden and looked after as family pets."

Cade's first experiment was to take urine from patients with schizophrenia, mania, depression, and normal controls and inject it into the abdominal cavity of guinea pigs. All the guinea pigs died. Cade believed that urea toxicity caused the deaths, so he decided to explore the influence of uric acid on urea toxicity. However, the uric acid was insoluble in water, and he could not inject it into the animals. To solve this, he used a soluble form of urate that had been known for at least 100 years and used as a treatment for gout (lithium urate). The posited toxicity of urea proved to be less severe in the presence of the lithium urate, so he next checked the hypothesized protective effects of lithium carbonate rather than lithium urate. The lithium carbonate also seemed to provide some protection against urea toxicity (Johnson 1984).

Cade (1949) decided to inject lithium into guinea pigs that he had not poisoned with urine to see what happened. The guinea pigs became placid for several hours and then returned to their usual frenetic behavior. Cade then experimented on himself to determine whether the lithium was toxic to humans and later tried the lithium on 10 patients with a range of diagnoses, including mania. Cade noted that the patients with agitation improved, but there was a considerable number of side effects and one patient died of lithium toxicity. Although unknown to him, Cade was retracing the steps of a Danish psychiatrist, Carl Lange, who had reached the same conclusions 50 years earlier and who had successfully given lithium to patients with affective disorders. Locked in the Danish language, Lange's work was not available to Cade. This caused an incorrect history of the "discovery" of lithium treatment that historians are finding difficult to resolve (for a translation of Lange's texts, see Schioldann 2001).

As discussed in Chapter 6, diagnosis and screening for hypertension was taking on a greater sense of urgency after World War II due to the skyrocketing incidence of cardiovascular disease. By the mid- to late-1940s, scientists had linked excess dietary sodium to hypertension, and primary-care physicians were recommending low-sodium diets for patients with this condition. Beginning in 1948, several companies began marketing lithium chloride (as opposed to table salt, which is sodium chloride) as a salt substitute. Lithium had been used as a table salt substitute throughout the nineteenth century for those on "low-salt" diets. In early 1949, reports of lithium toxicity began appearing in the lay press and in the medical literature about patients who had been using these salt substitutes. Eventually, the U.S. Food and Drug Administration (FDA) recommended that lithium salts should no longer be sold as a salt substitute. Notably, this marked one of the first tests of the FDA's jurisdiction because lithium salts were sold as a food and not a drug. Thus, the medical profession and the public already knew about the dangers of lithium, including death, before Cade's 1949 paper on treating agitation with lithium. Overcoming the fear of lithium toxicity would take decades.

One of the controversies within psychiatry involved a decade of debate about the efficacy of lithium in depression prophylaxis. The principle combatants were Michael Shepherd and Barry Blackwell in the United Kingdom and Mogens Schou and Poul Baastrup in Denmark. Schou and Basstrup advocated using lithium in the prophylaxis of depression, which doctors had done in continental Europe from about 1968 onward. Opinion leaders in the United States and the United Kingdom delayed lithium's use until a decade later. Shepherd and Blackwell had published a critique of Mogen's and Schou's original study describing evidence of lithium's effectiveness in preventing the relapse of depression. Over the next 10 years, these teams engaged in a protracted public-speaking, letter, and editorial campaign that ended only when Mogens and Schou presented results of a double-blind, placebo-controlled trial. However, the entire episode exposed how difficult it is to interpret data and scientific evidence for psychiatric illness. It also exposed the influential role of conceptual frameworks, in that excellent scientists could look at the same data and come to different conclusions. Schou summed up this controversy as follows:

To the nonpsychiatric bystander it must have caused astonishment that views so much in contrast to each other could be held by reputable psychiatrists. Even in the profession the debate generated concern, because it revealed a lack of solid knowledge about fundamental aspects of a supposedly well-known psychiatric disorder. It is presumably no coincidence that the protagonists in the debate, were, respectively, psychiatrists of the Kraepelinian school with its emphasis on manic-depressive disorder as one of the endogenous psychoses, and psychiatrists trained in the school of Aubrey Lewis, where stress is laid on the clinical continuity between depressions precipitated by a clear-cut external event and depression where such an event is less obvious but may still be suspected. The latter group of psychiatrists is more likely than the former to give strong weight to psychological factors and placebo controls. The debate served to highlight important unanswered questions. (Quoted in Johnson 1984)

Lithium eventually won FDA approval in the 1970s, although using it to prevent unipolar major depression remains controversial. Primary-care physicians who have less trepidation about prescribing other potentially toxic drugs (e.g., tricyclic antidepressants, anticoagulants, nonsteroidal anti-inflammatory drugs, among many others) only rarely assume the responsibility of initiating and monitoring of lithium. To a certain extent, this is because patients with mania and manic depression are relatively rare in primary-care practices. Others have suggested that lithium has no champions among pharmaceutical representatives (Shorter 1997). In terms of treating or preventing depression, primary-care physicians typically turn to the drugs with which they are more familiar, and later studies suggested that other antidepressants were effective for prophylaxis. Although doctors shunned lithium for years in both the United States and the United Kingdom, the story of the next class of medications is noteworthy for its differential adoption in the two countries.

The Story of Monoamine Oxidase Inhibitors

Germany initially bombarded London during World War II by using bombs dropped from airplanes. Later in the war, the German military delivered these bombs using jet rockets launched from the other side of the English Channel. They powered these V2 rockets, or buzz bombs, with a fuel consisting of liquid oxygen and ethanol. As supplies of these propellants ran low, the rocket engineers resorted to using hydrazine as a new substitute fuel. At the end of the war, there was a large and inexpensive supply of the hydrazine. Investigators studied derivatives of hydrazine for their potential usefulness against tuberculosis (Healy 1997; Le Fanu 1999). Hydrazine was already a desirable compound because the chemical companies that had been producing it for war were now reentering the peacetime marketplace. The success of drugs like the anti-malarials, penicillin, and streptomycin in treating human diseases demonstrated the pharmaceutical industry's remarkable potential. One derivative of hydrazine produced in 1951 in the United States was iproniazid, which scientists found to be effective against tuberculosis; physicians still use another such derivative, isoniazid, to treat tuberculosis today.

Clinicians treating patients with tuberculosis began to note that patients became euphoric, even though they were still ill from the tuberculosis. The euphoric side effects of iproniazid were so apparent that it fell out of favor as a treatment for tuberculosis (Healy 1997). Multiple investigators began testing the hypothesis that the drugs might be useful for patients with mental illness in general and depression in particular. While at least three or four groups were working on this hypothesis at the same time, Nathan Kline at Columbia University is credited with establishing the therapeutic efficacy of monoamine oxidase inhibitors for the treatment of depression.

Kline and his team reported that iproniazid resulted in mood improvement among some of their most chronically ill and functionally impaired patients on the psychiatric "back wards." This work, combined with the work of others, established monoamine oxidase inhibitors as effective drugs for treating depression. Kline pursued these findings with determination because the pharmaceutical company initially did not support this new indication. The drug had been developed for tuberculosis, and the company had reasonable concerns about the drug's toxicity. In a presentation at the American Academy of Neurology in 1958, Kline and Saunders (1959) made comments that typified their public relations campaign to get the appropriate backing for iproniazid:

The hepatotoxic effects of Marsilid (iproniazid) are at present restricting the rational use of this drug by those clinicians who do not look at the facts. Marsilid is unique, and no replacement is available.

The history of science is not simply the history of discoveries and new ideas that tend to approach closer to reality. It is also the history of the defense of these findings against errors due to propaganda, politics, and bureaucracy.

Soon after winning the needed support, doctors found that the drug caused jaundice in some patients, and regulators withdrew it from the market. Other monoamine oxidase inhibitors followed, but patients had trouble with headaches and elevated blood pressure. Scientists attributed these problems to the "cheese effect"—an interaction between the monoamine oxidase inhibitors and a chemical found in cheese and other foods (tyramine) caused the headaches. Providers also reported drug–drug interactions between monoamine oxidase inhibitors and commonly prescribed medications. Then in a clinical trial conducted by the Medical Research Council in the United Kingdom, scientists showed that phenelzine was no better than placebo in treating depression. Unfortunately, the dosage of phenelzine used in the Medical Research Council trial was too low; furthermore, it did not include sufficient subjects with phobic and atypical depression, the clinical subcategories for which phenelzine is most effective.

Companies marketing other antidepressants deliberately highlighted the side effects of the monoamine oxidase inhibitors. Although doctors in the United Kingdom still use monoamine oxidase inhibitors, doctors in the United States, especially those in primary care, use the drugs much less often. It is not clear why there was a differential adoption of the monoamine oxidase inhibitors in the two countries. Scientists and policy makers on both sides of the Atlantic had access to the same research data on effectiveness and side effects. For whatever reason, British physicians and patients found the risk-to-benefit ratio of the monoamine oxidase inhibitors acceptable, while American physicians and patients did not. This is noteworthy because it demonstrates how factors other than research data played an important role in the use of psychoactive medications. Nonetheless, some historians mark the monoamine oxidase inhibitors as the beginning of specific medications for depression. Others begin the story with the discovery of chlorpromazine, which led to imipramine and the tricyclic antidepressants.

The Story of Chlorpromazine

Paul Charpentier, a chemist in the pharmaceutical industry during World War II, investigated a series of phenothiazines for antimalarial activity. These agents are derivatives of methylene blue that Paul Ehrlich had demonstrated to have antimicrobial properties many years earlier (Healy 1997). The phenothiazines were not effective antimalarial compounds, but they did have properties similar to antihistamines. Henri Laborit, a French military surgeon, began working with antihistamines as an adjunct in anesthesia to prevent cardiovascular shock. Researchers discovered antihistamines in 1937 and evaluated them for treating psychoses, with negative results. Laborit began experimenting with the antihistamines for the anesthesia application as early as 1949, but with only limited results. In 1951, he noted that a newly synthesized antihistamine, chlorpromazine, functioned as a potentiator of anesthesia. He also noted that it resulted in patients displaying an "uninterest" in their surroundings. Although his subsequently published paper was about the drug's potential application in anesthesiology, he also reported that the drug could have applications in psychiatry. Soon after this, in 1952, Jean Delay and Pierre Deniker began testing the drug in patients with mental illness and reported surprisingly positive results. By the end of 1953, the drug was in widespread use in psychiatric hospitals in both the United States and the United Kingdom.

From the perspective of primary care, general practitioners are no more likely to initiate an antipsychotic for patients with schizophrenia than they would be to start lithium for patients with mania. Nor would they typically prescribe ECT for a patient with major depression or chemotherapy for a patient with breast cancer. Yet most primary-care physicians have prescribed chlorpromazine or related compounds to treat nausea. Primary-care physicians were still awaiting a safe and effective drug for patients with mild to moderate psychiatric illness.

In a small asylum in Switzerland in 1955, psychiatrist Roland Kuhn was investigating a drug similar to chlorpromazine for treating schizophrenia. Although the drug was chemically similar to chlorpromazine, it made the patients more agitated. A team of experts from psychiatry and the pharmaceutical industry hypothesized that the drug might have a euphoric effect. Kuhn and his team therefore decided to try it on patients with depression and found that patients with certain forms of depression made impressive improvements (Healy 1997). Kuhn proved that the new drug, imipramine, was an effective antidepressant, and it was the first of the tricyclic antidepressants. However, the pharmaceutical company did not aggressively market imipramine for this indication and remained ambivalent about whether there was a large enough market of patients with depression who might benefit from the compound. Kuhn's original article (1958) was hardly enthusiastic, as he recommended the drug only to treat "simple endogenous depression." He reported that outcomes were poor when mania, schizophrenic features, organic brain disease, epilepsy, and agitation accompanied the depression. Kuhn commented that "every complication of the depression impairs the chances of successful treatment."

Scientists also viewed the time lag between starting imipramine and the clinical response as another unacceptable limitation. As late as 1960, researchers were even studying imipramine combined with fever therapy to overcome the time lag (Lehmann 1960). Healy (1957) suggested the pharmaceutical industry's interest in imipramine ignited through two factors. First, an influential shareholder had a depressed family member successfully treated with the drug. Second, the company leaders saw the growing interest generated by the monoamine oxidase inhibitors.

The stories outlined above address just a few of the many compounds that scientists investigated for psychopharmacological action in the period between 1940 and 1970. We limited the accounts to those compounds that eventually proved important in the practice of psychiatry. Investigators also tested amphetamines, methylphenidate, antihistamines, chloral hydrate, morphine, adrenergic blockers, mescaline, adrenaline, and LSD, among a legion of other compounds for psychiatric applications (Rudolf 1949; Stunkard 1950; Himwich 1958). During the next few decades, many other psychopharmacological agents would follow, but the pattern of discovery, marketing, and clinical adoption followed the same model as that demonstrated by the examples provided in this chapter and the last.

Students of the history of these discoveries have adjudged the process differently, depending on their ideological stance on psychiatry in general. Take, for example, the summary statements of various analysts:

We have seen, however, that so far in the field of psychopharmacology, practice has outstripped theory. Though we recognize that tranquilizers correct certain schizophrenic symptoms, there is less agreement on the mechanism by which the improvements are achieved. Whether or not drugs effect cures is a problem for the future. But the practical value of the advance should not be underestimated. It may be compared with the advent of insulin, which counteracts symptoms of diabetes without removing their cause. (Himwich 1958)

Even if we think that many of the millions of sufferers from anxiety all over the world should preferably be treated on analytic couches, by individual psychotherapy, in therapeutic groups, by alteration of what is so often an unalterable environment, it is by the use of drugs and other simple and practical physical treatment methods that the vast majority are actually going to have to be treated in practice. (Sargant 1967)

It is one thing to demarcate an area for development, another to build prematurely on uncertain foundations. And it is indisputable that while the gap between established knowledge and much psychiatry theory and practice remains uncomfortably wide, there has been an understandable but nonetheless mistaken tendency on the part of some psychiatrists to traffic in uncertain assumptions, unfounded speculations, and unproven hypotheses which in some quarters have invested their role with the mystique of a priest or shaman equipped with the qualifications of an emotional engineer. Not the least of the disadvantages associated with an oversell of this type is the inevitable disillusion and resentment that follow on unmet claims and promises and that can exercise an adverse influence on development of the less spectacular but more solid work in progress. (Shepherd 1976)

This revolution was not so much worked towards as stumbled upon—and by chemists with no special interest in psychiatry and researchers who were looking for the answers to questions that had nothing to do with psychiatry. (Stone 1997)

This is a story of ambiguities and ideologies. The promise of a pharmacological scalpel that the antidepressants brought to psychiatry and the rise of a biological language that they gave rise to, looked at from a different angle, can appear little more than a cloak of artistic verisimilitude for quite other processes. (Healy 1997)

Post-war psychiatry had indeed been a "smashing success," but it is also deeply enigmatic. The "triumph" of human reason in understanding the neuroses—psychoanalysis—has been shown to be a sham, while the accidental discovery of the drugs "that really made a difference" were made completely independently of any intellectual understanding of mental illness. (Le Fanu 1999)

It is imperative to note that there is no evidence that those who developed these medications expected their widespread use in primary care. Chlorpromazine, reserpine, lithium, monoamine oxidase inhibitors, and imipramine did not open a new chapter in the history of the primary care of emotional disorders. The role of the early antidepressants in the care of patients in primary care was ambiguous until the 1980s. The following excerpts from an article providing "a guide for the general physician" demonstrate this confusion:

Choosing the most suitable antidepressive drug for the individual patient is not easy. This is not surprising when one considers that a given psychopathologic matrix may give rise to a variety of clinical symptoms. Furthermore, we have few reliable or easily useable diagnostic aids, either physiologic or psychometric, to help determine which of the available pharmacologic agents is indicated. And since we also know very little about the modes of action of the various antidepressants, it is remarkable that we do as well as we do. It should be remembered, too, that many depressive disorders—particularly those occurring in individuals who have a basically strong personality—are self-limiting. Physicians, being human, tend to credit the treatment in use at the time for the patient's recovery. This may help account for the high percentage of improvement reported in the vast majority of depressed patients regardless of the nature of treatment. (Schielle and Benson 1960)

The article went on to provide practical suggestions about choosing among sedatives, monoamine oxidase inhibitors, imipramine, electroconvulsive therapy, and combination therapy. The authors described these medications as symptomatic treatment, rather than as specific treatment of an underlying pathophysiology. The lack of diagnostic categories and the lack of a conceptual framework to guide physicians' choices of specific medications impeded the widespread recognition and treatment of depression in primary care. Researchers needed to produce evidence that doctors should use specific drugs to treat specific psychiatric illnesses. They also had to teach primary-care physicians a language and taxonomy that would identify emotional disorders as specific varieties of psychiatric illnesses.

This raises the issue of whether varieties of depressive illness are to be considered as "natural kinds" (i.e., as different species of orchids or different types of stones), all endowed with a fixed ontology and hiding out in the world ready to be discovered once and for all, or whether they are language constructs resulting from negotiations between "experts" and complainants. According to this latter model, nothing can guarantee the long-term stability of the varieties of depression, not even the fact that in the future they may be related to specific brain sites. This latter model implies that (*a*) clinical profiles of mental disease in general and those of the depressions in particular have "expiration dates" that in each case are determined by the rate of change in their biology and sociology; (*b*) not basic scientists but clinicians, whether generalists or specialists, are the real reckoners and narrators of disease; and (*c*) descriptions and classifications of depression constructed in general practice and in secondary or tertiary referral venues may be different but both are correct (Berrios 1994).

Summary

The goal of this chapter is not to make judgments about the theoretical underpinnings, efficacy, or appropriateness of antidepressant therapy or to impugn or celebrate the various players' genius or motives. We recount this history to show how it intersects with the story of reinventing depression in primary care. The new pharmacological agents opened a new chapter in psychiatry that started as early as the 1950s. We stress, however, that these agents changed psychiatry and treatments for those with severe mental illness. These new drugs did not change the care of mild to moderate emotional disorders in primary care; the drugs that changed the care of emotional disorders in primary care came not through psychiatry but through the pharmaceutical industry.

8

"PERFECT DRUGS" FOR PRIMARY CARE

As discussed, primary-care doctors and their patients have been using psychoactive medications to treat emotional symptoms for at least a century. Over the past 100 years, the toxicity and addictive properties of these drugs have improved, and the manner in which these drugs are discovered, tested, marketed, distributed, and regulated has changed. Antidepressant drugs are less revolutionary when viewed in the context of this history. This chapter tells the story of drugs used in the nonspecific treatment of emotional disorders in primary care since World War II, highlighting the limited role of the primary-care and psychiatry leadership in promoting and regulating the use of these drugs.

Brave New World

Aldous Huxley, the author of *Brave New World*, was born in Surrey, England, in 1894. Several of his family members suffered from depression, and his older brother's suicide at the age of 25 shattered Huxley's adolescence. The brother had gone walking on the grounds of a psychiatric hospital where doctors were treating him for depression and killed himself in the nearby woods (Bedford 1987). Aldous Huxley was deemed unfit for service in World War I because of his eyesight, and he lost several of his friends to the new form of mechanized battle. Huxley published *Brave New World* in 1932, between the two world wars. Although reviewers have considered the primary themes of *Brave New World* to express an anti-utopia and the tension between art and science, there is also a third theme: fear of Americanization (Bradshaw 1994). American values of mass production, standardization, capitalization, individualism, and consumerism bombarded Europe in the 1920s. *Brave New World* not only foretold a world where people traded personal liberty for self-gratification, but a world economy dominated by American ideals.

The leadership in Huxley's *Brave New World* did not maintain its power through violence, but through brainwashing and conditioning. One of its chief methods of assuring conformity was the drug "soma." Huxley (1994) described the development of soma as follows:

Two-thousand pharmacologists and biochemists were subsidized in AF 178 [178 years after Henry Ford]. Six years later it was being produced commercially. The perfect drug. Euphoric, narcotic, pleasantly hallucinant. All of the advantages of Christianity and alcohol; none of their defects. Take a holiday from reality whenever you like and come back without so much as a headache or a mythology. Stability was practically assured. It only remained to conquer old age.

Notably, Huxley penned these words well before the discovery of the modern arsenal of psychotherapeutic drugs, but obviously not before the time of alcohol, opium, bromides, and anticholinergics (such as scopolamine). Thus, while it is tempting to remark on the prescience of the potential for drug-induced conformity, it is also true that the notion of "an opium of the masses" is an age-old concern.

Huxley took the name "soma" from a drug with similarly claimed psychoactive properties mentioned in Native American folklore (Huxley 1959a). In Native American folklore, the drug had greater potential for adverse effects, including death. Huxley's later writings would return several times to the double-edged sword that psychotherapeutics offered: He saw both the potential dangers of chemical tyranny and the potential for treating psychiatric illness. He also wrote about the potential of using hallucinogens as a pathway to greater perception and insight. Thus, by the mid-1950s, he was a cultural icon in both the United States and the United Kingdom on matters ranging from pacifism to the balance between art and science to psychotherapeutics.

In January 1959, the University of California–San Francisco sponsored a three-day symposium entitled "A Pharmacologic Approach to the Study of the Mind." Many top U.S. scientists involved in new developments in psychopharmacology attended, and Aldous Huxley was the after-dinner speaker (Huxley 1959b). The attendees spoke with much excitement about the potential ability of drugs to alter specific components of brain chemistry, and to do so safely. Robert M. Featherstone, who made the opening remarks at the symposium, commented:

In anesthesia, one must maintain a particular level of central nervous system depression below the level of consciousness without disturbing the vital processes of respiration or circulation. However, [psychopharmacology] involving the effects of chemical compounds on the brain while maintaining consciousness is, I believe, a most fascinating approach to pharmacology and will be one of the most interesting in which we have ever indulged. (Featherstone and Simon 1959)

Although the attendees discussed the therapeutic roles of chlorpromazine, reserpine, and the monoamine oxidase inhibitors, they also considered the use of these medications (as well as lysergic acid or LSD, among others) as laboratory tools to investigate how the mind worked. Indeed, the possibility that these drugs might elucidate the workings of the mind was at least as exciting a prospect in 1959 as their therapeutic potential. A corollary of this prospect was the idea that differential responses to drugs might help resolve confusion in diagnostic criteria. In other words, an individual's response to a drug would help determine what disease he or she was suffering from. Were this true, investigators could develop objective diagnostic tests for psychiatric illnesses. This would overcome some of the shortcomings of diagnostic criteria based on patients' ability to communicate their subjective feelings and physicians' ability to label their symptoms. Scientists now recognize that it is wrong to infer diagnosis from response to treatment; this fallacy is called the "affirmation of the consequent."

The title of Huxley's (1959b) main talk at the San Francisco symposium was "The Final Revolution":

The Final Revolution, as I see it, is the application to human affairs, both on the social level and on the individual level, of technology. Now what is technology? Technology, technique in general I suppose, is the application in a perfectly conscious and rational way of well thought out methods of doing things efficiently. The watchword is "efficiency."

Huxley suggested that science's primary aim was to gain maximum efficiency by balancing human capacity with the capacity of technology. Huxley warned scientists of the dangers of sacrificing personal liberty and individual freedoms for the goal of efficiency and about the potential misuse of psychotherapeutics. He also warned the group about the hazards of conducting its work without adequate input from the community. As we describe later in this chapter, these warnings were prescient.

Finally, Huxley was the only participant to raise the issue of the increasing use of minor tranquilizers and the growing role of pharmaceutical companies. He complained that Wallace Laboratories had taken "soma" as the name of one of its new sedating compounds. We stress that scientists meeting at symposiums of experts on psychopharmacology, such as the one held in San Francisco in 1959, were not addressing the needs of patients with emotional disorders in primary care. None of the participants in the symposium represented primary care. Primary-care physicians did not use lithium, reserpine, monoamine oxidase inhibitors, or chlorpromazine in the care of patients with mild to moderate emotional disorders. Rather, psychiatrists used these medications to treat severe mental illness, and basic scientists used them to explore the brain's biochemistry. In 1950, primary-care physicians prescribed benzodiazepines for common diagnoses, such as psychoneurosis, anxiety, and psychosomatic illness. The idea of prescribing a specific drug for a specific emotional disorder was not a feature of the day-to-day practice of primary-care medicine.

Penicillin for the Blues

The first of the new drugs to change the prescribing patterns in primary care for the enormous population of patients with mild to moderate emotional symptoms was meprobamate, which had been discovered by Frank Berger, a Jewish refugee who fled from the Nazis. Berger demonstrated that meprobamate induced muscle relaxation and reduced anxiety while not producing sleep or addiction. Following the pattern repeated by several other drugs, Wallace Laboratories overlooked meprobamate and erroneously judged that no market existed for such a drug (Shorter 1997). Berger successfully promoted the drug, despite the company's ambivalence, and it named the new drug Miltown after the town in New Jersey that was its home. By the late 1950s, meprobamate became one of the most widely prescribed drugs in the world (Blackwell 1973; Montagne 1991; Shorter 1997). Primary-care physicians in both the United Kingdom and the United States made "Miltown" a household name and part of the cultural lexicon:

> Within two years of its introduction, meprobamate was all the rage, more of a cultural phenomenon than a significant medical advance. It was called the "penicillin for the blues"; an appropriate metaphor since the antibiotics, the exemplars of the "magic bullet" concept of pharmacotherapy, were still a wonder to the general public. Relaxing was called "miltowning," and mixing meprobamate with a Bloody Mary was referred to as a Miltown Cocktail. The drug's name became ubiquitous in societal discourse. It was the topic of conversation at coffee klatches and garden club parties in expanding suburbia. (Montagne 1991)

Meprobamate became one of the most widely prescribed drugs in primary care, but not for long. Other pharmaceutical companies took note of Miltown's unprecedented and unforeseen success and began marketing competing drugs. For the first time, the companies recognized the enormous pool of people who sought care for mild to moderate psychiatric symptoms and insomnia. Miltown died, but meprobamate did not. Rather, Wallace Laboratories began marketing meprobamate as "Soma." The generic name for Soma is carisoprodol, and it is still available by prescription as a muscle relaxant.

Another Jewish refugee from World War II, Leo Sternbach, was working in the pharmaceutical industry, searching for any substances with activity similar to meprobamate among the preexisting compounds at his disposal (Sternbach 1978; Shorter 1997; Le Fanu 1999). All were dead-ends, so in 1957, after three or four years of effort, his supervisors closed down the project, and Sternbach (1978) began retooling for another research program:

The working area had shrunk almost to zero and a major clean-up operation was in order. My co-worker, Earl Reeder, drew my attention to a few hundred milligrams of two products which had not been submitted for pharmacological testing at the time so we submitted them for pharmacological evaluation. We thought the expected negative result would complete our work."

Unknown to Sternbach and his team, one of the compounds had undergone a chemical change while sitting on the laboratory shelf. Animal testing on this implausible and unplanned derivative demonstrated its impressive potential to relax without sedating (Berrios 1983). The new compound, which laboratory workers could have just as easily tossed in the trash, became the first benzodiazepine, chlordiazepoxide. Chlordiazepoxide overtook meprobamate as the most frequently prescribed drug in primary care. Sternbach's subsequent discovery of diazepam, or Valium, in 1969 replaced chlordiazepoxide as the most prescribed drug.

In the early 1970s, Valium became the most commonly prescribed drug in the world, and it maintained this position for nearly a decade. The use of minor tranquilizers for treating mild to moderate emotional symptoms in primary care became a global phenomenon (Balter et al. 1974). Dunlop (1970) suggested that the drugs were so widely prescribed that the number of prescriptions "represents sufficient tablets to make every tenth night of sleep in the United Kingdom hypnotic-induced." Parish (1971) reported that 80% of all psychotropic drug prescriptions in the United Kingdom were for hypnotics and tranquilizers, while 7% were for stimulants, and only 14% were for antidepressants. For such a fundamental change in the drug treatment of emotional symptoms in primary care, one might have expected general medicine or psychiatry professional societies or academic research centers to have played a major role in leading the new treatment model. This was not the case, however. Local primary-care physicians, their patients, and the pharmaceutical industry championed the supremacy of minor tranquilizers in treating emotional problems in primary care with little input from the academic community or regulatory bodies.

Reports on how frequently people used these drugs sent shockwaves through the National Health Service. Parish (1971) commented:

It is necessary not only to examine psychotropic drug prescribing rates, patterns, and trends, but also the indications for their use. These can only be determined by relating treatment to morbidity. Unfortunately, such information is not available, and what information there is on the extent of psychiatric morbidity alone is most unreliable because of observer bias, differing parameters, confused nosology, and lack of replicability.

Parish was lamenting the fact that physicians prescribed these medications for a wide range of nonspecific symptoms and controversial indications. Using these drugs for indications other than those for which they were approved could be considered overuse or misuse.

In the United States, the pattern of use was much the same. In 1972, diazepam was the most commonly prescribed drug in the country, and chlordiazepoxide was the third most commonly prescribed drug. Physicians wrote more than 70 million prescriptions for these two drugs alone, at a cost of $200 million. In contrast, tricyclic antidepressants accounted for only 11% of all psychotropic drug prescriptions in 1972 (Blackwell 1973). In a U.S. national survey conducted in 1970–1971, the investigators reported that 22% of men and 37% of women had used either a prescription or a nonprescription psychotherapeutic drug in the past year (Parry et al. 1973). Diazepam maintained its position as the most frequently prescribed drug in the United States for six consecutive years between 1972 and 1979 (DeNuzzo 1979).

What explained the rapid and seemingly unimpeded diffusion of minor tranquilizers into so many Anglo-American homes? There was no large-scale educational campaign by any professional medical or psychiatric organization in an attempt to improve the recognition and treatment of emotional disorders in primary care. There was no multi-site clinical trial enrolling primary-care patients with criteria-based disorders and monitoring outcomes with standardized measures of severity. There was no health-services research demonstrating improved work productivity. There were no disseminations of screening instruments for emotional disorders, no practice guidelines, and no emotional disorder clinics. There were no national campaigns for anxiety awareness to facilitate help-seeking behaviors, no web pages for emotional distress, and no massive distribution of government-produced educational pamphlets. Academic psychiatry, academic medicine, mental health advocates, and governments were bystanders in this phenomenon for an entire decade. Instead, popular demand fueled the phenomenon of minor tranquilizer.

Even with the evidence of massive sales of minor tranquilizers, it is unclear whether the total intake of psychotropic medications in the community increased in the 1970s (Gabe and Williams 1986; Gabe 1991). For example, we do not know to what extent the increase in prescriptions for minor tranquilizers was offset by a decrease in the intake of barbiturates, alcohol, scopolamine, nicotine, major tranquilizers, and other psychotropic medications. A large percentage of the adult population had access to a bottle of pills but only used the drug intermittently as a safety net or as an occasional sleeping aid (Parry et al. 1973). In the United States, "mother's little helper" entered the lexicon as a socially acceptable way to get relief from day-to-day hassles, and middle-aged women became popularly identified as the primary users of tranquilizers, even though most users were older adults—65 years of age or older (Bury 1996). While it remains debatable whether the worldwide consumption of all psychoactive substances increased, the worldwide use of both prescription and nonprescription psychotropic medications did become concentrated within a single therapeutic class (minor tranquilizers) and, to a certain extent, within a few brand names (Valium and Librium).

Marketing Drugs in a Therapeutic Vacuum

There are at least three reasons why the minor tranquilizers became the predominant psychotropic medications: safety, efficacy, and marketing. Primary-care doctors did not use the drugs described in Chapter 7 because the experts had recommended them only for patients with severe mental illness. Using these drugs included not only the risk of side effects but also the risk of labeling a patient with a mental illness. Physicians and patients felt that labeling a patient with a nervous condition was different from labeling a patient with mental illness. Indeed, nervousness requiring a tranquilizer became a status symbol rather than a stigma. Primary-care doctors and patients viewed the risks of minor tranquilizers as almost nonexistent, both in terms of side effects and leaving a stigma. Thus, there was no effective braking mechanism to attenuate the tranquilizers' popularity, except perhaps for the cost of the prescription.

Primary-care physicians not only touted the minor tranquilizers as safer than the alternative, barbiturates, but they believed that they were a more specific treatment for "anxiety" (Berrios 1999a). Minor tranquilizers were more specific in that they were less sedating but still anxiolytic (i.e., they reduced the patient's anxiety symptoms). At the same time, they were the first drugs for which the primary-care community had received the "green light" from the psychiatric community as an appropriate drug therapy for their considerable population of patients with anxiety, psychoneurosis, and neurotic depression. One might argue whether psychiatry communicated a green light or failed to communicate a red light, but, in either case, physicians in general practice viewed the minor tranquilizers as safe and effective. In comparison, the psychiatric community had labeled the barbiturates, sedatives, and tonics in widespread use in primary care until 1955 as useless, dangerous, and addictive. However, while it had censured the available choices in the past, psychiatry suggested no practical alternatives; thus, the minor tranquilizers filled an enormous therapeutic vacuum.

Experts view meprobamate as the first "designer drug" in psychiatry because it was a product of the pharmaceutical industry (rather than academia) and because it responded to consumer demand. It was not the first psychoactive drug to become part of the popular culture: Alcohol, opium, heroin, cocaine, nicotine, and LSD, among others, have all played on this stage. However, meprobamate and diazepam probably enjoyed the most explosive and extensive worldwide distribution. There is no question that one of the major reasons for this explosion is that primary-care physicians could repeatedly see, with their own eyes, that the medications filled an important unmet need for their patients (Horder 1991). The patients relayed their satisfaction with the medications not only to their physicians but also to their friends and family; physicians relayed their satisfaction with the drugs to other physicians, and so on.

It would be interesting to know how much of the "snowball rolling downhill" phenomenon of minor tranquilizers would have occurred even without the marketing blitz financed through both paid advertising and the popular press. We will never know because pharmaceutical companies spent an enormous amount of money in the 1970s and 1980s on marketing. Advertisements appeared in professional journals and through mailings to physicians, while pharmaceutical representatives visited with primary-care physicians face to face. J. E. Prather (1991) reported there was one pharmaceutical sales representative for every 8 physicians in the United States and for every 18 physicians in the United Kingdom. In 1960, when chlordiazepoxide overtook meprobamate in sales, physicians received

forty separate direct mailings, in addition to long playing phonograph records (a novelty in 1960) containing physicians' testimonials of wondrous drug results. Eight page advertisements appeared in leading medical journals. When Valium was featured in more advertisements in medical journals than any other prescription drug (1972–1977) Valium became the most widely prescribed drug in the world. (Prather 1991)

The marketing of minor tranquilizers reached such a frenzy that sociologists, psychologists, and marketing students began studying pharmaceutical companies' promotional techniques. Critics charged that these promotional campaigns created an image that medicalized common, everyday hassles and stresses. These marketing techniques and the perceived overuse of these medications eventually resulted in a divisive backlash and massive debates on both sides of the Atlantic. The debates concerned a variety of issues, including whether the drugs worked at all, whether regulatory bodies had failed to protect the public (Mintz 1965), and whether common human qualities had become "mystified." These concerns were not limited to popular press outlets. Consider this condemnation from *Science* magazine:

It is apparent that the pharmaceutical industry in redefining and relabeling as medical problems calling for drug intervention a wide range of human behaviors which, in the past, have been viewed as falling within the bounds of the normal trials and tribulations of human existence.

Changing the human condition is a monumental undertaking. While seeking to change cognitive shapes through chemical means is more convenient and economical, the drug solution has already become another technological Trojan horse. (Lennard et al. 1970)

In both the United States and the United Kingdom, academics convened symposiums to consider the implications of the widespread use of minor tranquilizers in the 1970s. Government agencies commissioned expert committees and held official hearings, and regulatory bodies met to consider new guidelines and sanctions. The media ran stories of innocent people who had become hooked on the drugs. Scientists published new studies exposing the potentials for abuse and addiction. Sociologists examined the evidence of disproportionate use by gender, race, and class distinctions, while psychologists provided testimony that the drugs might impede true healing and problem solving. Most important, society began to view the users of these drugs as no different from those abusing alcohol, marijuana, and cocaine. In 1973, Parry and colleagues described the debate as the "Invention of Happiness versus Pharmacologic Calvinism":

There are opposing—and often extreme—views being taken on the use of psychotherapeutic drugs. One combines permissiveness and very high expectations for smooth daily living and may well stem from one of the main streams of our cultural history. The French revolutionary St. Just once boasted, "We have invented happiness." Like many such inventions, it may have originated in Europe but it came into mass production in the United States, coupled with the expectation that life could, indeed should, be free from care and stress. The corollary of this demand for happiness as a right and an end in itself often is an unwillingness (or even inability) to tolerate "normal" discomfort and malaise coupled with the belief that to grin and bear it is less a sign of moral strength and virtue than it is a sign of stupidity or lack of sensitivity. To many members of this school of thought, psychotherapeutic drugs—at least the more common varieties—are simply adjuncts of comfort and utility.

The opposing view—equally extreme—is based on another thread of our history—the puritanical view of life. In the field of psychotherapeutic drug use, it manifests itself in what Klerman has aptly called "pharmacologic Calvinism." It is this school of thought that, in its popular manifestation, paints a gruesome picture of an overmedicated society, perpetually swallowing tranquilizers to escape from the relatively mild and almost universal troubles that man is born to and thus undermining social character. Sometimes the charges appear in more modern populist guise: behind the overmedicated society are gullible physicians pushed into overprescribing by the machiavellian marketing techniques of the pharmaceutical industry.

These fundamental debates about the role of psychoactive medications in treating emotional disorders in primary care demonstrate that social norms may dictate that a treatment is unacceptable even if it is scientifically sound and readily available. Unfortunately, the arguments about the role of minor tranquilizers occurred in a context in which there was little or no science on their proper role in primary care.

Decision-Making in an Evidence-Based Vacuum

One of the most surprising aspects of the rise of the minor tranquilizers and the subsequent debate on the proper treatment of anxiety and neurotic depression is an absence of any discussion of the underrecognition and treatment of depression before the 1980s. The antidepressant drugs unquestionably lost the battle for primary-care physicians and patients at least until the middle of that decade. Academic psychiatry failed to convince primary-care physicians to treat specific psychiatric diseases and not simply emotional symptoms. Primary-care doctors failed to lead research in their own practices to better understand the proper role of the drugs they prescribed most often.

In the United States, the number of prescriptions for minor tranquilizers rose from 40 million in 1964 to 90 million in 1972. Over the same period, the number of prescriptions for antidepressants per year rose only from 10 million in 1964 to 18 million in 1972 (Blackwell 1973). It is important to recognize there was no consistent authoritative expert voice against using minor tranquilizers in primary care. Indeed, physicians could have readily gone to the mainstream medical literature at this time and produced dozens of articles that purported to provide evidenced-based recommendations on the appropriate use of minor tranquilizers in primary care. In addition to their patients telling them that the medications worked, as well as their own observations that their patients' functioning had improved, the primary-care physicians could point to expert recommendations. These recommendations suggested that primary-care physicians rely on expert clinical judgment. Writing in the *Journal of the American Medical Association* in 1973, Blackwell commented:

Surprisingly little research has been carried out to define the nature of psychiatric conditions in general practice. The emotional disturbances in these patients is uncertain, though it is known that the large preponderance of mental disorders either alone, or complicating physical disease are of a minor or neurotic nature.

It is still less clear how these minor emotional disturbances in general practice should be classified. The words anxiety or depression are often applied alone or in combination to describe a range of emotional experiences. The semantic confusion and symptomatic overlap is profound, with some evidence that suggests that the names used to describe the illnesses are chosen to reflect the drugs available to treat them.

In the United Kingdom, there was no consensus regarding the widespread use of these drugs. In 1972, the U.K.'s Department of Health and Social Security sponsored a symposium entitled "The Medical Use of Psychotropic Drugs" (Parish 1973). Organizers convened the symposium to discuss the widespread use of these drugs and the steps leaders should take to reduce their use, but participants reached no consensus. While Parish and Dunlop seemed to view the rates of use of these medications as unimpeachable evidence of misuse, other commentators were more ambivalent. For example, Margot Jefferys (1973) suggested:

We should remember, however, that human beings consume many other products which also affect the mind but which we do not label medicine and which are available to a greater or lesser extent without medical sanction, for example, alcohol, tobacco, coffee, tea, and marijuana.

One advantage of the fact that the National Health Service funds prescription medications is that it can monitor prescription drug use. In the early days of opium, bromides, and barbiturates before World War II, no nation had this capacity. Thus, the extent to which people consumed these medications before the 1950s is undocumented. Physicians dispensed many of these drugs from their offices without recording the transactions. Many other psychoactive drugs were routinely available without a prescription. The ability to monitor the use of prescription drugs requires not only that there be drugs available only by prescription, but also that there be a centralized authority interested in monitoring expenditures for these drugs. With computers, this monitoring capacity became increasingly cost-effective. Thus, minor tranquilizers became available when regulatory agencies could monitor their distribution. In the United Kingdom, because the National Health Service covered prescription drugs, the rising cost of these medications was a major factor in reviewing their use.

The discussion at the U.K.'s Department of Health and Social Security symposium ended in a stalemate: The attendees did not reach a consensus on whether the widespread use of minor tranquilizers signaled misuse. However, the conference did provide a platform upon which to lament the lack of a workable diagnostic classification scheme for emotional disorders in primary care. A. M. W. Porter, a general practitioner participant, commented that "in the field of affective illnesses, the whole subject of classification seems to be in a dreadful muddle and it is no consolation to reflect that this situation has now persisted for more than 40 years" (Parish 1973). As late as the 1980s, leaders in primary care continued to voice such criticisms:

Drug therapy has change remarkably in content but less remarkably in volume. We appear to prescribe as many modern psychotropics now as we did barbiturates and bromides in the 1950's. . . . A major problem with psychiatry in general and with general practice psychiatry in particular is that the conditions and situations encountered exist as descriptive collections largely of symptoms and a few signs with little correlation with any substantive pathological or biochemical changes. (Fry 1982)

Even within the psychopharmacology community, there was no agreement about the specificity of the new drugs for particular affective disorders. In 1959, William Malamud listed four possible therapeutic results from psychotropic drugs:

1. Results that are primarily symptomatic in that they influence beneficially undesirable clinical manifestations of a given illness
2. Results that are produced by interfering with the course of the pathophysiological processes caused by the disease
3. Results that are produced by the elimination of primary causative factors
4. Results that are produced by prevention of disease.

Malamud concluded that psychopharmacological agents acted via the first-listed mechanism: They improved symptoms but did not attack the underlying cause of the disease. For example, a patient may take an antihistamine for a runny nose, while recognizing that the medication will not cure the viral illness that caused the runny nose. No virus-specific treatment is available, so there is no reason to diagnose the specific virus. This argues against the need for diagnostic specificity because there was no therapeutic specificity. In the case of emotional symptoms, if a physician's treatment options are the same for cause A and cause B, there is little reason to make the effort to distinguish between the two. Nearly 40 years

later, Healy (1997) made similar arguments regarding the currently available armamentarium of psychopharmacologic agents.

Consider the ambivalent and mixed messages sent out to primary-care physicians by the *Journal of the American Medical Association* in November 1964. In
the November 2 issue, Jonathon Cole, the head of the Psychopharmacology Research Center at the National Institute of Mental Health, wrote a review on antidepressants at the request of the American Medical Association's Council on
Drugs. After reviewing more than 70 controlled trials, Cole opined:

Unfortunately, despite the controlled studies reviewed in this paper and the much larger
number of uncontrolled studies available in the literature, it appears impossible at this time
to define specific types of depressed patients for whom a given specific drug is clearly indicated.

In mild depressions, conservative or supportive management with or without the use of
a sedative tranquilizer, such as meprobamate, deprol, or chlordiazepoxide is worth trying
initially since spontaneous improvement may occur, and these agents carry the least risk
that unpleasant or dangerous effects may occur.

Three weeks later, in the November 23 issue of the *Journal of the American
Medical Association*, Nathan Kline published a review on the practical management of depression in conjunction with his 1964 Albert Lasker Clinical Research
Award for the discovery of monoamine oxidase inhibitors. In his acceptance lec-
ture, he stated:

For the practical purpose of an acute treatment the classification of the depression is usually unimportant.

A depression without psychological or situational justification is classified as a psychosis even if mild, and even if the patient is clear mentally. Such a psychotic depression is
almost always easier to treat than the neurotic one which usually requires a psychiatrist.

Ideally, the decision as to which antidepressant to use should depend upon the condition
of the patient, but as previously indicated the classification of depression is unsatisfactory
and there is no way to decide which of the two groups of antidepressants is better for a particular use.

Thus, opinion leaders in specialty psychiatry were endorsing the basic nonspecific treatment approach that primary-care physicians used to treat mild emotional
disorders. These statements indicated that sedative-hypnotics and anxiolytic
agents were reasonable first choices in treatment. There was no suggestion that
specific antidepressant drugs were available for specific diagnostic categories.

There was no consistent voice suggesting that primary-care physicians should
not use the minor tranquilizers, and there was evidence that these agents were
more effective and less toxic than the tricyclic antidepressants in the treatment of
neurotic depression. As early as 1969, D. Wheatley reported a comparative trial of
imipramine and phenobarbital in depressed patients enrolled from general practices in the United Kingdom. He concluded that "[our] results are in agreement
with a number of those quoted, failing to demonstrate any advantage for imipra-

mine over phenobarbitol in these cases of neurotic depression." Writing in the *Proceedings of the Royal Society of Medicine* in 1972, Wheatley reported on eight years of experience in conducting similar randomized trials in a consortium of general practices in the United Kingdom. He designed these trials to test several of the sedative-hypnotics, minor tranquilizers, and antidepressants. Wheatley again concluded that anxiolytic drugs were more effective in neurotic depression. L. E. Hollister, writing a general review on antianxiety and antidepressant drugs in the *New England Journal of Medicine* in 1972, was equally ambivalent about the efficacy of the antidepressants. He cited several studies showing no improvement over placebo. Then, writing in the *Journal of the American Medical Association* in 1973, Blackwell summarized that

patients of general practitioners with anxiety-depression syndromes do as well or better when receiving minor tranquilizers compared to tricyclic antidepressants. . . . Not only are the tricyclic antidepressants no more effective than the anti-anxiety drugs in most illnesses, but the latter are safer.

Thus, on both sides of the Atlantic and as late as the mid-late 1970s, the message received by primary-care physicians was this: Psychiatric diagnostic categories for emotional disorders are at best subjective and probably irrelevant. The data suggested that primary-care physicians could use benzodiazepines successfully, safely, and symptomatically for most of the emotional problems seen in primary care. These doctors were hearing from their patients that the drugs worked and from the pharmaceutical companies that the medications had a broad range of clinical indications (Horder 1991).

The Strident Voice of Psychiatry

Although about 10% to 20% of psychotropic drugs prescribed in general practice were antidepressants, P. Tyrer (1978) found that "general practitioners are using antidepressant drugs in inadequate dosage on a large scale. If antidepressant drugs are being prescribed nationally in a similar dosage to those in this study they are being given as sedatives rather than antidepressants." Until the mid-1980s, psychiatry-based knowledge and recommendations regarding the appropriate diagnosis and treatment of affective disorders were peripheral to the practice of primary care. Specialty psychiatry's advice to primary-care physicians was frequently condescending and impractical. Psychiatrists with no record of research or clinical experience in primary care offered recommendations for primary-care physicians. Furthermore, these experts often disagreed among themselves. Although the reviews of Kline and Cole (mentioned above) serve as two examples, we offer two additional examples.

William Sargant—as discussed, a champion of physical methods of treatment in psychiatry—was an early critic of using antidepressants for severe depression.

Sargant favored the more conventional treatment, ECT. Sargant (1961) presented a paper on the drug treatment of depression to the Annual Meeting of the British Medical Association in 1960, sharing his view that

large numbers of [patients committing suicide] are just depressed patients who have already been seen by doctors and who have obtained so very little help from them that suicide seems the only way out of their problems and suffering. . . . In the large numbers of treatable cases of depression being seen by general practitioners and physicians everywhere the diagnosis may be overlooked for long periods of time. . . . To put deeply depressed patients on imipramine alone, and to have them too long on it while awaiting possible improvement, may actually result in a marked worsening of symptoms and in what should have been a quite unnecessary suicidal attempt.

Various psychiatric experts repeated similar comments innumerable times in the medical literature over the next 30 years, often decrying primary-care physicians' poor clinical acumen. These types of pronouncements, made in ignorance of the types of psychiatric problems most often seen in primary care and in denial of the diagnostic and treatment debates within the psychiatry community, have been counterproductive. Indeed, 40 years later, there have been no randomized trials demonstrating a reduction in suicide mortality via early recognition and treatment of depression in primary care, and suicide reduction has not been used as an outcome measure in antidepressant drug trials.

Moving from the ambiguous to the impractical and from the United Kingdom to the United States, Frank Ayd, an early psychiatrist leader in psychopharmacology and in developing and testing tricyclic antidepressants, wrote a monograph on recognizing and treating depression that he specifically targeted to general practitioners. In the 135-page work, the author devoted 114 pages to the presenting symptoms, recognition, and diagnosis of depressive disorder; 10 pages to patient education; and only 8 to 10 pages to drug treatment (Ayd 1961). Ayd's recommendations emanated from a wealth of clinical experience, but, unfortunately, none of this clinical experience was based in primary care. Furthermore, the finer points of these recommendations relied heavily on judgments about the specific subtypes of depression. As psychiatry experts had already communicated to primary-care physicians, the subjectivity of these assessments was unacceptable, even among experienced psychiatrists diagnosing severely mentally ill patients.

Ayd recommended barbiturates as a sleeping aid for those patients with mild depressions and admonished general practitioners that "fewer mistakes will be made with antidepressants and more favorable results will be achieved if they are not prescribed for every type of depression, but reserved for those patients for whom they are indicated." Using unstandardized and unblinded outcome assessments, Ayd reported mixed outcomes with 30% of patients improved, 48% partially improved, and 22% unimproved at two months. He reported noncompliance (now for some incomprehensible reason called "nonadherence") and minor side effects as common problems. Thus, while suggesting that "therapy must be tailored to the needs of the individual depressive," psychiatry was unable to communicate the practical details of its recommendations to its own rank and file, let alone the primary-care community.

This comment by M. M. Weissman and G. L. Klerman as late as 1977, in a journal unknown to primary-care physicians, using data from their own specialty practice, and communicated to and about community psychiatrists, typifies this problem:

It is our impression from our own clinical and research experience that the failure to recognize depression at diagnosis is coupled with extensive reliance on minor tranquilizers of the meprobamate and diazepoxide series and other sedative-hypnotic agents. In contrast, the tricyclic antidepressants are probably underutilized and there is a discrepancy between the findings of clinical trials and prescription practices in these patients.

Community-based psychiatrists were also prescribing the minor tranquilizers at a high rate and often failing to diagnose depression, especially chronic depression. In another study that highlighted the limited diffusion of new advances in psychiatry to the psychiatric community, M. B. Keller and colleagues (1982, 1984) reported findings from the National Institute of Mental Health Collaborative Study on the Psychobiology of Depression. The results of this study were disturbing because the participating centers in this multi-site study were all clinical programs in specialty psychiatry (as opposed to primary care). Keller and colleagues reported that most patients treated in the community for depression had not received adequate treatment. Psychiatrists treated many patients with anxiolytic medications such as benzodiazepines, and among those patients treated with antidepressants, the prescribed dose was usually too low. Even more surprising, Keller reported inadequate treatment at the five academic centers participating in a clinical trial:

We examined the treatment of 338 patients with nonbipolar major depressive disorders during the first eight weeks after entry into the National Institute of Mental Health–Clinical Research Branch Collaborative Program on the Psychobiology of Depression: Clinical Study. Of the 250 entered as inpatients, 31% received either no antidepressant somatotherapy or very low or unsustained levels, and only 49% received at least 200 mg of imipramine hydrochloride (or its equivalent) for four consecutive weeks. Of these patients, 19% received less than 30 minutes of psychotherapy per week. Among the 88 who entered as outpatients, 29% received no antidepressant somatotherapy; another 24% received very low or unsustained levels; only 19% received at least 200 mg of imipramine hydrochloride or its equivalent for four consecutive weeks. Of these patients, 52% received less than 30 minutes of psychotherapy per week. (Keller et al. 1982)

Keller and colleagues (1984) also found that 21% of the patients treated at these academic psychiatry units failed to recover after two years of care. This study provided direct evidence that not only had recent advances in treating depression failed to reach primary-care physicians, even psychiatrists at academic medical centers were unable to reach targeted levels of treatment. The authors concluded that "more research is needed to determine how patients and practitioners contribute to this phenomenon of low intensity of somatic treatment."

The Absent Voice of Primary Care

Between 1955 and 1980, academic psychiatry offered platitudes but no practical advice for primary-care physicians. Primary-care physicians and their leadership played the role of pawns. Although primary-care practitioners' research on the clinical epidemiology of psychiatric illness appeared as early as the 1950s, the practitioners failed to translate their data on prevalence into treatment recommendations or outcomes research. There were, of course, isolated exceptions, such as Wheatley's work, but these efforts were neither widespread nor coordinated. The voice of general practitioners was absent regarding the appropriate use of benzodiazepines and the development of other recommendations for treating emotional disorders in primary care. The few recommendations that general-practice leadership did endorse were treatment suggestions they had adopted from specialty psychiatry.

The tendency of specialty psychiatry, patients, policy makers, and the media to vilify general practitioners for their role in the perceived overprescription of the minor tranquilizers makes the absent voice of general practice even more disturbing. Recall that, in the mid- to late-1970s, when these criticisms had reached their peak, cost and time concerns had already begun to erode patients' confidence in their primary-care physicians. It was a short leap of logic to assume that doctors used the minor tranquilizers to get patients out of the office quickly without dealing with their problems in a substantive manner:

Indeed, the willingness of various specialists openly to criticize others in the medical field, and to be outspoken about the pharmaceutical industry, set the scene for wider public disquiet. One of the main lines of argument put by influential hospital-based psychiatrists and psychopharmacologists, particularly in the early phase of the debate about the overuse and misuse of the drugs, was that general practitioners had been remiss in their prescribing behavior.

In making these claims, medical critics were also revealing and exacerbating longstanding divisions within the British medical profession, albeit ones that were also usually hidden from view. . . . The historic division between hospital specialists and general practitioners, in Britain, has often led to conflict within the profession as a whole. In the case of hospital psychiatrists, the debate about the benzodiazepines broke out at a time of renewed crisis for the psychiatric profession, as it tried to fashion a new role for itself within a fast changing health care system. . . . Not surprisingly, therefore, when patient and consumer groups took up the issue of the benzodiazepines, they also directed some of their fire at general practitioners. (Bury 1996)

We find little evidence that primary-care physicians and their leaders openly acknowledged the problem or aggressively participated in solving it until people outside primary care activated a significant social movement. Patients believed that their advocacy was the proximate cause of new regulations and safeguards

(Lader 1996; Bury 1996), taking the view that these safeguards would never have occurred with primary-care physicians providing the leadership.

There is some evidence that patient concerns about the lack of adequate protection from psychoactive medications and the poor teamwork between psychiatry and primary care have not been forgotten. Lader (1996) suggested that

patients have become more reluctant to take tranquilizers. They no longer seek them out as the answer to their psychological and bodily symptoms. Indeed, they are reluctant to take any psychotropic medication, questioning the need for, and the addiction potential of anti-depressants.

The benzodiazepine controversy balkanized the primary-care psychiatry landscape. Psychiatry, primary care, patients, advocacy groups, regulatory agencies, pharmaceutical companies, insurance companies, academia, and private practice were all in separate camps. This is the landscape in the early 1980s:

Though some people in medicine, and in the pharmaceutical industry, may feel that caveat venditor should now be their watchword, as they face mounting challenges, especially from the media and from consumer groups, it needs to be recognized that medical controversies, such as that over the benzodiazepines, often arise from divisions among medical experts themselves. Far from presenting a "united front" to the outside world, practitioners in medical science and medical care have become more divided, as expertise and specialization have grown, and as different interest groups have flourished. Under these conditions expertise fractures, and expert knowledge becomes, in the sociologist Anthony Gidden's phrase, "chronically contestable." It is in the gaps produced as a result of such "contests" that media and popular campaigns have taken root. From the scientific viewpoint, lay ideas and "beliefs" have been seen as largely irrational and epiphenomenal. The social configuration of health and illness in modern societies makes this outlook increasingly untenable, as moral and political values become caught up with health disorders. (Bury 1996)

Bury's comments were remarkably consistent with Huxley's warnings in 1959 quoted at the beginning of this chapter. The more we blur the boundary between disease and normal human behavior, the more likely it is that society will question the values of science and demand a role in forming policy. Primary care has become the focal point, if not the flashpoint, for these debates because this is where most people seek care for their symptoms and concerns. Frank Ayd (1961) echoed William Sargent's 1960 expectation that by 1985 "there should be no case of emotional illness that cannot be treated by the general practitioner." By the end of the twentieth century, that expectation still had not become reality.

Summary

Between 1960 and 1985, the nonspecific provision of minor tranquilizers dominated the treatment of emotional disorders in primary care. Patient demand, safety, effectiveness, and marketing all stimulated the widespread nonspecific prescription of these medications. Psychiatry and primary-care leaders were not important participants in the diffusion of these new medications. Neither did psychiatry and primary care collaborate effectively to improve the care of patients with emotional disorders. The data are ambiguous in regard to the question of whether the total intake of psychotropic drugs actually had increased. The perception that these drugs were over- and indiscriminately prescribed resulted in a much closer monitoring of the treatment of emotional problems in primary care. This monitoring emanated from the public's demand and only secondarily spread to the psychiatry and primary-care leadership.

Through the 1980s, benzodiazepines were prescribed less frequently, and diagnoses of anxiety, neurotic depression, and psychoneurosis began to diminish. Physicians began to prescribe antidepressant medications for depression. This new treatment paradigm for emotional disorders, arising in the 1980s, remains the dominant model today. Unlike the advent of anxiety and anxiolytics, specialty psychiatry, the National Institute of Mental Health, consumer groups, and both community-based and primary-care-based research played a role in developing, implementing, and promoting the new paradigm.

Accomplishing this sea change in primary care required a platform supported by four major pillars:

1. A substantial overhaul of the diagnostic criteria for emotional disorders.
2. A method to measure the severity of illness and how it changed over time with treatment.
3. A biomedical framework for the pathophysiology of depression that dovetails with the specific mechanism of how antidepressants work.
4. A better understanding of the clinical epidemiology of emotional disorders in primary care.

We discuss each of these four pillars in the following chapter. While these pillars were developing to some extent between 1950 and 1980, they did not result in a stable platform for treating emotional disorders in primary care until the late 1980s.

9

THE BIRTH OF THE CURRENT
TREATMENT PARADIGM

The current treatment paradigm for depression in primary care has existed for only about a decade, and developing it involved many researchers and a great deal of funding. It was invented through research in psychiatry and stimulated by an ever-growing awareness of the public health effects of depression. In this chapter, we describe the four pillars of the new model: *(1)* new diagnostic criteria for emotional disorders, *(2)* new measures of severity, *(3)* a disease-specific biomedical framework, and *(4)* a better understanding of the clinical epidemiology of emotional disorders in primary care. We emphasize that the model is relatively new, based on the best available evidence, understood as incomplete, and expected to change.

The Untamed Wilderness of Psychiatric Classification

During much of the nineteenth century, St. Louis, Missouri, served as the point of departure for explorers, traders, and settlers heading out into the vast, untamed territory between the Mississippi River and the Pacific Ocean. In a similar way St. Louis became the point of departure for the westward expansion of psychiatric diagnosis in the late twentieth century. Standardizing psychiatric diagnosis was viewed as a major step toward taming the wilderness of subjectivity and unreliability in psychiatric classification (Berrios 1999b). The initial goal had been to provide explicit diagnostic criteria that would guide researchers. However, the process of bringing science to the art of psychiatric diagnosis raised considerable controversy among those who viewed these developments as contributing to the reification, americanization, and medicalization of psychiatric illness.

Furthermore, these criteria quickly crossed the boundary between research and clinical practice and then crossed the Atlantic Ocean to influence both European research and subsequent revisions of the World Health Organization's International Classification of Diseases (Pinchot 1997). Eventually these criteria would influence decisions about health-care policy, third-party payments, professional privileges, and the social boundaries of mental illness. These criteria are important because they define who is sick. Such criteria are inherently controversial and involve both scientific and social concerns. Debate about the boundary between mental illness and mental health is longstanding, as this quote from the nineteenth century suggests:

In considering the actions of the mind, it should never be forgotten that its affections pass into each other like the tints of the rainbow; though we can easily distinguish them when they have assumed a decided color, yet we can never determine where each hue begins. (Ferrier 1824)

Before the 1980s, explicit diagnosis of emotional disorders in primary care was simply not a recognized component of the standard of care. Instead, between 1945 and 1980, primary-care doctors had treated emotional problems based on their patients' most troubling symptoms. Patients and the broader society were comfortable with the language and social construction of "nerves" or "anxiety" or "insomnia." Because effective drugs were available to treat these symptoms, doctors treated patients either with reassurance or with the latest available sedative or anxiolytic. Between 1945 and 1980, the available sedative changed from bromides to chloral hydrate to barbiturates to benzodiazepines, but the basic treatment paradigm was essentially the same. In addition to the external backlash against psychopharmacology amid the benzodiazepine controversy, there was also growing criticism about the efficacy of psychoanalysis and embarrassing data about the variability in psychiatric diagnosis. It became clear that psychiatry could not move forward if its leaders, researchers, and practitioners did not even share a common language.

As late as 1980, psychiatric researchers at different academic centers within the same country did not communicate well with each other, and clinicians working in the same hospital did not reliably assign the same diagnosis to each individual patient. A series of research studies from the 1950s to the 1980s documented a situation in which primary-care physicians lacked an appropriate framework for diagnosing explicit emotional disorders before prescribing diagnosis-specific treatments.

In the 1950s, researchers began testifying to the unacceptable state of psychiatric diagnosis (Beck 1962). For example, Pasamanick et al. (1959) analyzed the psychiatric diagnoses given to 538 women admitted to three different but comparable wards in a psychiatric hospital in 1956 and 1957. The researchers found that doctors systematically differed in the rates at which they applied various diagnostic labels and that they used different treatments for the different diagnoses. The team concluded:

Despite protestations that their point of reference is always the individual patient, clinicians in fact may be so committed to a particular psychiatric school of thought that the patient's diagnosis and treatment is largely predetermined. Clinicians . . . may be selectively perceiving and emphasizing only those characteristics and attributes of their patients which are relevant to their own preconceived system of thought. This makes it possible for one psychiatrist to diagnose nearly all of his patients as schizophrenic while an equally competent clinician diagnoses a comparable group of patients as psychoneurotic.

In 1959, E. Stengel reviewed classification methods developed by psychiatrists in academic centers in multiple countries and then interviewed clinicians regarding their perceptions of existing classification schemes, as well as the current World Health Organization classification scheme for psychiatric diagnoses. C. A. H. Watts and Stengel prepared a report for the WHO's Expert Committee on Mental Health. Their summary comments provide a general view of the state of psychiatric diagnosis at mid-century:

Everybody who has followed the literature and listened to discussions concerning mental illness soon discovers that psychiatrists, even those apparently sharing the same basic orientation, often do not speak the same language. They either use different terms for the same concepts, or the same term for different concepts, usually without being aware of it. The lack of a common classification of mental disorders had defeated attempts at comparing psychiatric observations and the results of treatment undertaken in various countries or even in various centers of the same country. (Watts and Stengel 1966)

In addition to unclear definitions of concepts, other investigators demonstrated that clinicians were susceptible to subjective influences, their environment, and prior labels when making diagnoses. For example, M. K. Temerlin (1968) played an audiotape of a psychiatric interview with a normal individual to three groups of psychiatrists and psychologists. He allowed one group to "overhear" that an expert believed the patient was psychotic, while another group "overheard" an expert suggest the patient was healthy, and a third group heard neither of these comments. Both "overheard" diagnoses had a significant influence on the likelihood that the respondents would choose the sham diagnosis. Notably, the psychiatrists were more susceptible to the overheard inference than the clinical psychologists were. Even those clinicians who had chosen not to endorse the diagnosis they had overheard gave the presumably healthy individual a wide range of diagnoses.

Another study demonstrated that psychiatric diagnoses also varied among countries. In 1968, M. G. Sandifer and colleagues filmed 30 patients undergoing clinical interviews in a North Carolina psychiatric hospital. The research team played these films for groups of psychiatrists in North Carolina, England, and Scotland. Not only did the investigators find important differences in diagnoses among countries, but also psychiatrists within the same country had difficulty with achieving consensus. Psychiatrists in all three countries viewed the same videotape of the same interviews, yet British psychiatrists diagnosed manic depression more frequently, while U.S. psychiatrists were more prone to diagnose neurotic depression, and the Scottish psychiatrists tended to diagnose personality disorder. Clearly, these psychiatrists had been reacting to patient cues and prioritizing symptoms in ways that resulted in different psychiatric diagnoses.

Other studies have demonstrated these different diagnoses as well. Beginning in the early 1970s, R. E. Kendell and colleagues (1971) reported the results of several studies emanating from the United States–United Kingdom Diagnostic Project. The first study employed methods similar to those in Sandifer's videotape study. The research team showed eight videotapes (five English and three American patients) to large audiences of psychiatrists in both the United States and the United Kingdom. Three of the patients presented classic symptoms, and the British and American psychiatrists largely agreed on these cases. They also agreed to some degree regarding three other patients, but the British psychiatrists were more likely to diagnosis affective psychosis. For the remaining two patients, they substantially disagreed, with the American psychiatrists tending to diagnosis schizophrenia and the British psychiatrists diagnosing personality disorders or neurotic illness. The authors commented:

In a situation such as this, where two groups of equally experienced psychiatrists, both provided with the same data, disagree as to whether or not a patient is schizophrenic there is a natural temptation to ask who is right. It is important to realize, though, that in our present state of knowledge such a question is not only unanswerable, it is inherently meaningless. . . . The decision whether or not an individual patient has schizophrenia can only be made by the "Hippocratic procedure" of comparing his symptoms with those of the illness and deciding whether the resemblance is adequate. . . . One cannot meaningfully discuss which is right for we have no external criteria to appeal to—no morbid anatomy, no etiologic agent, no biochemical or physiological anomaly.

The team also studied 250 consecutive admissions to a New York psychiatric hospital and a London psychiatric hospital. They found that rates of diagnosing various disorders differed between the two sites, but the differences largely disappeared when the scientists used explicit criteria. The group then compared diagnoses at nine state hospitals in New York and nine mental hospitals in London. Psychiatrists at New York hospitals diagnosed nearly 62% of their patients with schizophrenia, but those at London hospitals made the same diagnosis for only 34%. When psychiatrists used explicit criteria, their diagnoses of schizophrenia yielded rates of 29% and 35%, respectively. Similarly, overall, psychiatrists diagnosed depressive psychoses in 4.7% of the New York patients and 24% of the London patients, but when they used explicit criteria, the rates were 20% and

23%, respectively. This study provided unequivocal evidence that psychiatrists on both sides of the Atlantic were using different diagnostic criteria (Cooper et al. 1972; Kendell 1975). Again, these diagnostic differences resulted in treatment differences. Kendell (1975) suggested:

> The importance of the variations in diagnostic criteria that have been described here lies in the grave effects they are liable to have on communication. If different people use labels in different ways they will at best fail to communicate accurately, and may well actively mislead one another. The fact that American and British psychiatrists mean different things by schizophrenia, and probably have done for over thirty years, means that throughout this time each has been both misunderstanding and misleading the other. Awareness of the differences that previously went unrecognized also necessitates an extensive reappraisal by British psychiatrists of much American research, and vice versa.

Perhaps the low point for psychiatry in regard to the public's recognition of the shortcomings of psychiatric diagnosis came with the 1973 publication of a flawed (Farber 1975) but highly publicized study in *Science*, the premiere general scientific journal in the United States (Rosenhan 1973). Eight "sane" patients, most of whom worked in psychiatry or psychology, presented themselves to 12 psychiatric hospitals on the East and West coasts of the United States. All 12 gained hospital admission by complaining that they had heard voices saying "empty" or "hollow" or "thud." All reported that the voices had stopped, and all presented themselves otherwise as their "normal" selves. Doctors diagnosed seven of the "pseudopatients" with schizophrenia and one with manic-depressive psychosis and hospitalized them for 7 to 52 days. The author, Rosenhan, himself one of the pseudopatients, reported that other patients routinely recognized the pseudopatients as normal. He reported the important consequences of the early labeling of the pseudopatients as schizophrenic and suggested that the psychiatric hospital environment played an important role in reinforcing labels. Rosenhan refused to find fault with the clinicians, choosing rather to blame the system of diagnosing and treating psychiatric illness, as well as the destructive environment of the mental hospital.

By the mid-1970s, psychiatry was debating the merits of various extant classification systems, as well as whether diagnosis itself was useful at all. Such influential psychiatrists as Karl Menninger in the United States called for abolishing diagnosis in psychiatry (Menninger 1963; Kendell 1975). Menninger had laid out a cogent argument explaining that diagnosis was not only unreliable and invalid but also harmful because it labeled patients. Menninger argued that mental symptoms exist on a continuum and that patients differed only in the quantitative distribution along this continuum: "The discrete psychiatric syndromes about which Kraepelin wrote were conceptualized by Menninger as reducible to one basic psychosocial process: the failure of the suffering individual to adapt to his or her environment" (Wilson 1993). Emil Kraepelin, a nineteenth-century German psychiatrist, had designed a classification scheme based on longitudinal observations of patient course and prognosis:

Kraepelin's psychiatry became so influential because it offered a pragmatical, clinically and prognostically oriented nosology, developed by a self-confident author who focused on rather straight-forward quantitative and naturalistic research methods and claimed to abandon speculative aspects from psychiatry as much as possible. (Hoff 1995)

For Menninger, there was no clear demarcation between mental illness and health. Rather, there was a fluid boundary that any given individual could cross, depending on his or her adaptation to stress. This concept of a fluid boundary between mental health and illness also highlighted the importance of the cultural context in adjudging what is normal as opposed to abnormal behavior—"hence the answer whether an individual is mentally sound or not is ultimately determined by whether he has an integrated universe consistent within the given cultural framework" (Bertalanffy 1968).

Psychiatry was not alone in debating the threshold between disease and wellness. Consider an analogous controversy regarding essential hypertension in the early 1960s, as outlined by Sir George Pickering's research team:

The older view is that essential hypertension is a specific disease entity, and that subjects with and without the disease can be separated sharply on the basis of their arterial pressures. This hypothesis conforms to the general belief that disease represents a qualitative deviation from the norm. The new view is that essential hypertension represents a quantitative and not a qualitative deviation from the norm; that there is no natural dividing line between normal and abnormal pressures, and that any attempt to divide pressure sharply into normal and abnormal is artificial. (Oldham et al. 1960)

One could easily substitute "mental illness" for "essential hypertension," and this comment would capture the sentiment of Menninger and others. However, the essential hypertension debate did not become divisive, nor did it occur against the backdrop of a specialty in distress, as psychiatry was in the 1970s. Pickering and his group did not use their observations to suggest that diagnosing hypertension had no value; rather, they suggested that scientists base research and treatment recommendations on empirical evidence. Eventually, these observations led to George Rose's recommendations for both individual- and society-based approaches to cardiovascular risk factors.

One of the daunting problems in determining who has a mental illness is the lack of an objective criterion that observers outside of the patient can see and measure. Hypertension also exists along a continuum, and there is no clear demarcation of when the elevated blood pressure becomes a risk factor or a disease. Hypertension researchers, however, have the luxury of the sphygmomanometer—a device that can accurately measure the level of a person's blood pressure. During the 1970s, this led to the idea of "caseness." A case is someone who meets criteria for treatment. The idea was to construct a measure (e.g., a critical blood-pressure value) that respected a continuum between health and disease and offered various possible definitions of caseness. Although there might be some debate about the definition of a case, at least scientists could communicate their definition to other scientists in an objective manner. Psychiatrists did not have such a measure, and they argued about the need for such a classification scheme.

On the opposite pole from Menninger, other psychiatrists were calling for a return to a Kraepelin-type classification scheme. Psychiatry had gone so far in dismissing the necessity of explicit diagnoses that experts devoted entire texts to defending it (Kendell 1975; Rakoff et al. 1977). As Kendell remarked: "In most branches of medicine the value of diagnosis is never questioned. Its importance is self-evident because treatment and prognosis are largely determined by it." Other commentators recognized that the lack of an agreed-upon diagnostic classification scheme relegated psychiatry to the status of a nonscientific discipline:

Why make a diagnosis? Why not treat each patient as an individual apart from his diagnosis? The answer is that without diagnosis or categories or typologies we have no science. Perhaps this is what the anti-diagnosis people want—an unscientific floundering political field in which anyone with empathy, from ward maid to psychiatrist, from concierge to bartender to prostitutes, may be equal, and where "encounter" groups of any type may flourish. (Grinker 1977)

Whether arguing for a new diagnosis scheme or no diagnosis scheme at all, clearly, psychiatry could not avoid change. Unfortunately, the way forward was so murky and controversial that the field remained in limbo for a quarter century. Indeed, it is rare to read a history of psychiatric classification and diagnosis in which the author does not make the analogy to a "Gordian knot."

Given the chaotic state of diagnosis within the psychiatry community, primary-care physicians had to rely on a practical approach that focused on relieving presenting symptoms; consequently, screening for undiagnosed illness made no sense. Furthermore, many patients were benefiting from the symptomatic approach. According to Wilson (1993), a variety of factors resulted in cutting the Gordian knot:

In short, a confluence of pressures on the profession from outside influences—the major providers of resources for psychiatric research and treatment and the gathering momentum of the antipsychiatry critique—threw the issues of diagnostic reliability, treatment outcomes, and accountability for those outcomes into bold relief. Under these unfavorable professional conditions, the psychosocial model, as the dominant organizing model of psychiatric knowledge and the source of many of these problems, would have to be significantly altered—if not jettisoned altogether.

In other words, the profession perceived that it was losing prestige and research dollars, third-party payors did not know what they were paying for, and the public was uncomfortable with the ambiguous dividing line between mental health and illness. One of the profession's primary responses was to develop new measurement tools: criteria-based diagnostic schemes, measures of severity, and screening tools to identify psychiatric distress in large populations. In the following sections, we discuss how scientists developed each of the four pillars that provided a foundation for a new treatment paradigm for emotional disorders in primary care.

The First Pillar: Criteria-Based Diagnosis

Historians often regard the third revision of the American Psychiatric Association's Diagnostic and Statistical Manual (DSM) as the opening salvo in forcibly moving psychiatry toward a more scientific and medical model. Other experts have cited the work of researchers at St. Louis's Washington University as setting the stage for the medical model of psychiatry (Spitzer et al. 1978). Faculty in the Department of Psychiatry at Washington University published the "Feighner Criteria" in 1972, which constituted the first set of explicit and practical criteria for a limited number of psychiatric diagnoses to be used in psychiatric research. Researchers used the new criteria extensively in both the United States and the United Kingdom (Feighner et al. 1972). In the United Kingdom, Wing and colleagues (1974) developed a case-identification method using the Present State Examination, which provided an extensive list of patient symptoms based on 140 items. The researchers identified these symptoms with 38 possible syndromes and applied an "index of definition" to provide levels of confidence that symptoms were of sufficient severity to merit a diagnosis. Finally, the team applied a computer algorithm using the symptom data to make a tentative diagnosis based on terminology from the International Classification of Disease (ICD). On both sides of the Atlantic, researchers were working to increase the reliability and validity of psychiatric diagnoses, and eventually they teamed up to bring the DSM and ICD criteria closer together. By 1979, research teams were working on the Composite International Diagnostic Interview, which the World Health Organization adopted as the international standard in the 1990s (Wing et al. 1981; Robins et al. 1994). The following story focuses on the effect of the DSM-III.

The Feighner criteria became the predecessors of the Research Diagnostic Criteria in 1978, which were the predecessors of the DSM-III (Wilson 1993). The DSM-III, published in the early 1980s, changed the face and focus of psychiatry:

From the end of WWII until the mid-1970's, a broadly conceived psychosocial model, informed by psychoanalytic and sociologic thinking, was the organizing model for American psychiatry. As biologic insights into the nature of psychopathology accrued, the prefix "bio" was added to "psychosocial" to give use the now familiar "biopsychosocial" model. With the appearance of DSM-III, the essential focus of psychiatry shifted from the clinically-based biopsychosocial model to a research-based medical model. And through the development of DSM-III, research investigators replaced clinicians as the most influential voices in the profession. (Wilson 1993)

Wilson also described the political battles waged in developing the DSM-III and the substantial influence of social conventions, various special-interest groups, professional needs, and third-party payors' demands on formulating and defining diagnostic categories. For example, one controversy centered on the use of the term "neurosis." The developers rejected the terms "psychoneurosis" and "neurotic depression," mainstays of diagnosis in primary care (as well as clinical psychology) for the past 30 years:

There is no agreement in our field as to the generic name for an episode of serious depressive illness. We use the term "major depressive disorder" as it seems general enough to encompass the many further subdivisions that are the basis of much current research. This category includes some cases that would be categorized as neurotic depression, and virtually all that would be classified as involutional depression, psychotic depression, and manic depressive illness, depressed type. (Spitzer et al. 1978)

In defending these decisions, the same authors argued:

Neurotic depression is variously used to mean nonincapacitating, nonpsychotic, nonendogenous, nonrecurring, noninstitutional, nonbipolar, due to conflict, or some unspecified combination of all of these features. We believe that each of these features can be better studied separately than by combining them into a single class.

The Research Diagnostic criteria had specified subtypes of major depressive disorder, including primary, secondary, recurrent unipolar, psychotic, incapacitating, endogenous, agitated, retarded, situational, simple, and predominant mood. In addition, they included classifications for minor depressive disorder with significant anxiety, intermittent depressive disorder, panic disorder, generalized anxiety disorder with significant depression, phobic disorders, and obsessive-compulsive disorder. Not all of these categories and subdivisions survived the maturation process to the DSM-III, and not all have survived through subsequent revisions of the DSM. In addition, not all are included in the ICD. Not even the distinction between anxiety and depression has a clear demarcation (Johnstone et al. 1980; Roth and Mountjoy 1990).

Although scientists formulating a diagnostic classification scheme may have aspired to a scientific enterprise, the final product was clearly a social construction informed by partial data and accumulated clinical experience. Over the past 20 years and with subsequent revisions, Wilson noted that the conventions and language of the DSM are "being applied in daily teaching and practice and necessarily take on the look of something that, more and more seems natural—not made by human hands." From the perspective of primary care, it is important to realize the turmoil and uncertainty out of which this classification scheme arose and that the categories are actually just hypotheses regarding how emotional disorders might be distinct disorders, diseases, or entities. Nonetheless, in the United States and in many other countries, criteria such as DSM-IV (1994) became the mainstay of psychiatric diagnosis.

The Second Pillar: Severity of Illness

Mapping the boundaries of these hypothetical disorders required longitudinal studies of patient course and clinical trials of various therapies to determine whether there was any treatment specific to the posited disorders. However, if the field of psychiatry had a classification scheme by the 1980s, it still lacked a measure of severity in order to monitor symptoms over time. This quote from the methods section of a clinical trial in the 1940s highlights the problem:

The degree of depression present at the commencement of treatment is difficult to define accurately, but, with the exception of 3 cases treated at an outpatient clinic, it was sufficiently severe for all patients to be willing to pay specialist fees. (Rudolf 1949)

How do clinicians or researchers determine whether the severity of depression changes over time in response to therapy? In addition, how do they compare the outcomes reported for one treatment with those reported for a different treatment? With hypertension, a standard protocol for measuring blood pressure facilitates communication among researchers: moreover, each clinician has the same instrument readily available in his or her own clinical practice. We can measure glucose, cholesterol, hemoglobin, and white blood cells reliably and objectively, but we do not have a method to do this with pain and emotional symptoms. The dominant severity and change measures for anxiety and depression did not come from a team of psychiatrists, psychometricians, or statistical researchers at one of the academic psychiatric centers in the United States or the United Kingdom. Rather, a clinician-researcher working in relative isolation at a small mental hospital in England developed the measure that became the mainstay of clinical trials of emotional disorders.

During World War II, Max Hamilton was the Medical Officer in a Royal Air Force unit caring for men with combat fatigue. Many of these men had flown 30 or more bombing raids over Europe, but to discourage others from leaving duty for emotional problems, these men were labeled as having "lowered moral fiber" (Roth 1990). World War II offered many people the opportunity to rethink the boundaries of mental illness. Hamilton decided to pursue a career in psychiatry after the war and held various hospital positions in and around London. A lifelong interest and aptitude in mathematics led him to training in statistics and factor analysis. Clinical appointments with little research infrastructure, however, dominated his early career. In 1953, he developed an anxiety scale for a local trial of meprobamate and then in 1957, he developed a scale for depression, the HAM-D. Hamilton constructed the scale by subjecting detailed clinical features of hospitalized patients with depression to a factor analysis. By 1967, he combined further work on the depression scale with detailed instructions on how to administer it. Hamilton required that users make a clinical diagnosis, determine that the patient was free from physical disease, and ensure that final endorsements reflected observations by both the rater and a relative or nurse.

Hamilton originally designed the scale as a method to quantify a clinical interview: "The HAM-D was not meant to be a diagnostic scale but to measure what Hamilton called years later 'the burden of disease'. It was also meant to capture state rather than trait features—that is, phenomena susceptible to change" (Berrios and Bulbena-Villarasa 1990). By the 1970s, the scale was gaining acceptance as a standard scale of depression severity because it was concise, had acceptable reliability and validity, and measured a wide spectrum of depressive symptoms. By the 1980s, researchers regarded this scale as the standard scale to both select patients for clinical trials and measure change over time. The HAM-D also became the preferred measure of severity for the World Health Organization. Other scientists developed many other scales designed to measure severity of depression, but none has displaced the HAM-D. Part of this is because the HAM-D now has the weight of 30 years of common usage across multiple countries and languages, and its continued use makes it possible to compare more recent results with the extant literature. The importance of such a scale and its acceptability lies in the researchers' ability to test the efficacy of interventions compared with placebo or other treatments. It also enables researchers to compare outcomes across disparate interventions and clinical trials. Measurement in psychiatry remains a highly controversial area even after several decades of research on new instruments (Berrios and Markova 2002).

The Third Pillar: A Biomedical Model

By 1980, psychiatric researchers had the reproducible criteria needed to enroll homogenous groups of depressed patients in clinical trials and a reliable measure to record changes in the severity of symptoms with treatment. Innovations in clinical trial methodology and new methods of statistical analysis also had reached a new stage of maturation, as the randomized clinical trial became the gold standard of assessing the efficacy of a new treatment. This set the stage for rigorous clinical trials of antidepressants, psychotherapy, and anxiolytics in treating patients with major depression. One example of this research was the National Institute of Mental Health's Treatment of Depression Collaborative Research Program. In this study, 250 patients "were randomly assigned to one of four 16-week treatment conditions: interpersonal psychotherapy, cognitive behavior therapy, imipramine hydrochloride plus clinical management (as a standard reference treatment), and placebo plus clinical management" (Elkin et al. 1989).

Unfortunately, the study's results are difficult to interpret because the findings rely on the interpreter's frame of reference and how he or she analyzes the data. In a simple analysis of the outcomes of all four groups, there was no difference between any of the treatment assignments. At 16 weeks, subjects receiving the active treatments did about the same as subjects receiving clinical management plus placebo. In any number of secondary analyses, researchers drew different conclusions (Elkin et al. 1989, 1995; Imber et al. 1990; Shea et al. 1992). Nearly 20 years after the study began, experts still debate what it showed (Healy 1997). A clinician employing any of these four treatments could find evidence that his or her particular intervention was efficacious. In this sense, this was an important clinical trial because investigators demonstrated that doctors could treat depression. These types of studies contributed to the debate within psychiatry regarding the efficacy of psychotherapy and antidepressants, but they did little to change the treatment paradigm for emotional disorders in primary care.

By the late 1980s primary-care physicians generally accepted antidepressants as the most effective treatment. Whether the message was emanating from the National Institute of Mental Health, the pharmaceutical industry, or medical journals, primary-care physicians heard the consistent message that antidepressants were now the standard of care for depression. Psychiatry also provided general physicians and the public with a biomedical model describing the therapeutic specificity of antidepressants. For example, writing in *Science* in 1967, psychiatrists in the National Institute of Mental Health reported that

[previous studies] have shown a fairly consistent relationship between the effects of drugs on biogenic amines, particularly norepinephrine, and affective or behavioral states. Those drugs which cause depletion and inactivation of norepinephrine centrally produce sedation or depression, while drugs which increase or potentiate brain norepinephrine are associated with behavioral stimulation or excitement and generally have an antidepressant effect in man. From these findings, a number of investigators have formulated the concept, designated the catecholamine hypothesis of affective disorders, that some, if not all, depressions may be associated with a relative deficiency of norepinephrine at functionally important adrenergic receptor sites in the brain, whereas elations may be associated with an excess of such amines. (Schildkraut and Kety 1967)

Regardless of its accuracy, this catecholamine hypothesis provided physicians with a simple medical model of illness that they could present to their patients with depression. A debate about the efficacy of antidepressants was not a major barrier to treating depression in primary care. Both psychiatrists and primary-care physicians had some trepidation about primary-care physician's clinical abilities in diagnosing criteria-based depressive disorders and in managing treatment with tricyclic antidepressants. An editorial in the *British Medical Journal* summarized the questions emanating from primary care:

About one-fifth of the patients actually attending a family doctor's surgery are mentally disturbed and he undertakes the care of most of them. The commonest disturbances encountered are anxiety and depression. Their management raises questions of practical importance. How do they present? How can they be detected? How and by whom should they be treated? How effective is their management and how can it be improved? Unfortunately there have been remarkably few investigations into the clinical forms, natural history, and response to drugs and psychotherapy of affective illnesses in the setting of general practice. (Editorial [unsigned] 1970)

Anticholinergic side effects of the tricyclic antidepressants (e.g., dry mouth, urinary retention, sedation, and cardiovascular effects) were also a concern. Primary-care physicians already steered away from drugs like lithium, the monoamine oxidase inhibitors, and chlorpromazine because they viewed the side effects as unacceptable. Furthermore, in the mid- to late 1970s, criticism from many corners of society regarding primary-care physicians' perceived misuse of benzodiazepines was just reaching its peak.

Understandably, patients and physicians expressed concern that the antidepressants were just another class of medications being hailed as a "breakthrough." With time, doctors were concerned that these new drugs also would prove to be harmful. The biomedical framework, which identified the drugs' specificity, helped alleviate some of these concerns.

The Fourth Pillar: Epidemiology of Depression in Primary Care

Reinventing the treatment paradigm for affective disorders required new data on the clinical epidemiology of psychiatric illness in primary care, including prevalence, morbidity, and costs. Studies by Shepherd in the United Kingdom and Peterson in the United States described the prevalence of emotional problems and the standard of care in primary-care settings, relying on primary-care physicians' diagnoses (Peterson et al. 1956; Kessel and Shepherd 1962). In 1970, David Goldberg and Barry Blackwell, researchers in the department of psychiatry at the University of Manchester, published a study describing the prevalence of specific psychiatric conditions in a practice of general medicine. The study was unique in that the researchers compared the rate of psychiatric illness detected by the general practitioner, the study psychiatrist, and a symptom scale, the General Health Questionnaire (GHQ). The study found that about 20% of patients had psychiatric illness, mostly emotional disorders. The general practitioner missed one out of three of the cases. What made this finding remarkable is that the "general practitioner" was a trained psychiatrist who had only recently assumed the role of general practitioner and was fully aware of the study's goals:

Even though the general practitioner was himself an experienced psychiatrist, strongly motivated by the condition of the survey to detect emotional disturbances, he was not aware of one-third of the psychiatric disturbances. These cases of hidden psychiatric illness were just as severe as those recognized. What distinguished these patients is that the majority formulated their problems in somatic terms not only to the doctor but also to themselves.

The authors noted that only by direct questioning, either through the GHQ or a clinical interview, could or would these patients reveal their psychiatric distress. They also noted that patient–physician contact time was typically only 10 to 15 minutes and that most patients did have a medical diagnosis, as well as the psychiatric diagnosis. Over the next 20 years, numerous studies would report substantially similar findings.

In the United States, President Carter called for a Presidential Commission on Mental Health in 1977 to determine the population's mental health–care needs and to describe how and where providers delivered these services. As a preliminary answer to these questions, D. A. Regier et al. (1978) used data from multiple, existing surveys to piece together a picture of mental health services, demonstrating that most patients with mental illness who sought care received it in primary care. Furthermore, one in five patients with mental illness was receiving no formal care. Dubbed the "de facto U.S. mental health care system" the authors reported that in the United States 60% of those with mental illness were receiving care in primary care. About 21% did not receive care, 15% received care in a specialty mental health setting, and 4% received care as inpatients in general hospitals. Even though it was based on secondary data analysis, the study demonstrated that one important method to improve the quality of mental health care was to improve its delivery by primary-care physicians.

In 1980, Goldberg and Huxley (1980) summarized a decade of clinical epidemiology research in primary-care settings in both the United Kingdom and the United States, including the findings of Regier noted above. The authors reported that approximately 250 persons per 1000 in the community suffered from psychiatric illness in a given year. Of these 250 persons with psychiatric illness, primary-care physicians would see 230 persons for various presenting complaints but not necessarily for psychiatric illness. Of these 230 persons, the doctor would diagnose only about 140 as mentally ill. Among those recognized as mentally ill, psychiatrists would see only 17, and they would admit only 6 to a psychiatric hospital.

The new epidemiological data demonstrated a significant mismatch between patients needing mental health care and patients receiving this care. The mental health sector was caring for only about 15% of these patients. At least 20% were not even seeking care, but the overwhelming majority of patients at least had been seen in primary care during the previous year. The data also suggested that the quality of care for the common mental disorders seen in primary care was inadequate. Unfortunately, the data were still lacking on how inadequate it was and how to remedy the problem. These reports made it undeniably clear that providers could not improve mental health in the United Kingdom and the United States without improving the mental health care delivered in primary-care settings. The realization that primary care was the main provider of mental health care and that one in five patients with mental illness was receiving no care resulted in a shift of investigative interest to primary care and community settings. President Carter's Commission on Mental Health eventually led to the largest and most comprehensive national survey of the prevalence, incidence, and care of mental illness to date: the Epidemiologic Catchment Area Program, or ECA study. According to Wilson, the ECA resulted in a "needs assessment" for mental health and subsequently stimulated both research and education in primary care.

The United Kingdom provided early leadership in the epidemiology of emotional problems in primary-care settings. A national agenda for the next phase of research proved more difficult to formulate, fund, and activate, however. In 1984, the Institute of Psychiatry in London convened a conference on "Mental Illness in Primary Care Settings" (Shepherd et al. 1986). The organizers proposed three objectives for the conference: "First, to foster and deepen exchanges between researchers and policy-makers; second, to review the present lessons from research in this field, and third, to help construct a future research strategy which will assist policy decisions." The 150 attendees included researchers in primary-care psychiatry and representatives from nursing, social work, and psychology, the Department of Health and Social Security, the Medical Research Council, the Mental Health Foundation, and the World Health Organization. During the two-day conference, the attendees heard presentations and discussions regarding the current state of research and clinical care on mental health in primary care. The conference organizers also presented a research agenda outlining priorities for research and the funding that would be required to carry out this research. The proposed agenda focused on increasing research on treatment effectiveness, recognizing mental disorders in primary care, and improving training general practitioners in psychiatric skills. In general, the researchers communicated frustration with the lack of resources to carry out this agenda in the United Kingdom:

[The United States reported] an impressive list of existing and potential research work. It is perhaps paradoxical that an energetic research program is being fostered in a country with a comparatively chaotic and poorly developed primary care system, where research must be difficult. This contrasts with the position in the United Kingdom, where there are fewer barriers to research, but where we seem to be less highly motivated. (Cooper 1986)

The main component of the U.S.'s energetic research program to which Cooper had referred was the Epidemiologic Catchment Area study, which had already begun to produce results by 1984. Overall, 32% of Americans had experienced a criteria-based disorder at some time in their lives, 20% had an active disorder, and 15% suffered from the disorder in the past month. Only 19% of those with an active disorder had sought treatment in the prior 6 months. The study also found that 18% of the population, and 60% of those with at least one disorder, had met criteria for at least two psychiatric disorders in their lifetime (Robins and Regier 1991). For panic disorder, 91% of those with the diagnosis also had at least one other psychiatric diagnosis; the comparable rates for dysthymia were 86%, major depression, 75%, and phobia, 63%. The authors concluded that having one disorder placed the patient at risk for subsequent disorders. The study showed that the frequency of mental disorders was much greater than previously documented, that patients with these disorders often failed to seek care, and that most of those seeking care received it in primary-care settings. The investigators suggested:

If professionals in the general medical sector and social agencies are alerted to the association of mental disorders with work and marital problems, they can serve as detection, early treatment, and referral sources for those in need. To reach those with psychiatric disorders who are not in contact with medical and social agencies, a three-pronged educational program may be needed: (*1*) teach the public how to recognize these disorders, (*2*) inform them that many can be effectively treated, and (*3*) improve access to care.

Announcing a New Treatment Paradigm

In 1987, these findings and recommendations led to the National Institute of Mental Health's "Depression-Awareness, Recognition, and Treatment" (DART) program. This program's goal was to communicate to primary-care providers, mental health specialists, and the public that depressive disorders are common, serious, and treatable (Regier et al. 1988). The National Institute of Mental Health (NIMH) funded most of the program. Before initiating its training for physicians, NIMH convened a group of experts to review the state of the art in depression and to identify areas of scientific agreement regarding diagnosis and treatment. The group's consensus formed the basis of current diagnosis and treatment recommendations for the care of depressed patients. The program funded academic centers to develop short-term training programs on treating depression, focusing on primary-care physicians and psychiatrists. Finally, beginning in 1988, the program began an educational campaign aimed at the lay public, including radio, television, and print media advertisements. Locally, the organizers facilitated collaborative campaigns with local and regional mental health advocacy groups. Regier et al. (1988) suggested that this program was "the first major US public health prevention program targeted to a specific group of mental disorders."

In the United Kingdom, the Defeat Depression Campaign was initiated in 1992. Its three goals were to "educate health professionals, particularly general practitioners about the recognition and management of depression; educate the general public about depression and the availability of treatment in order to encourage people to seek help earlier; and to reduce the stigma associated with depression" (Paykel et al. 1997). Private sources funded the program, which was a joint effort of the Royal College of Psychiatrists and the Royal College of General Practitioners. The leaders published consensus guidelines on treating depression, offered training at national meetings for primary-care physicians, and conducted a public education campaign using multiple media outlets (Paykel and Priest 1992; Paykel et al. 1997). The organizers increased the content of psychiatric training for general practitioners, so that 40% of general practitioners spent six months in a psychiatric service during their clinical years. Paykel and colleagues (1997) noted that

expectations for such a campaign ought to be modest. The financial resources of the campaign were small, provided predominantly by donations from drug companies, other companies and organizations, and the Public Education Department of the Royal College of Psychiatrists.

In these campaigns, academic psychiatry in both countries communicated in a unified voice for the first time to mental health specialists, primary-care providers, and the public what constituted the standard of care for depression. Thus, the current treatment paradigm for emotional disorders in primary care emerged around the year 1990.

Summary

In the late 1970s, the fallout from the controversy over benzodiazepines left primary-care psychiatry in disarray. Specialty psychiatry leaders, primary-care physicians, mental health advocacy groups, and health-care policy makers were at best not communicating and at worst fighting among themselves. Reversing this state of affairs in the 1980s required the wholesale novel construction of a new treatment paradigm for depression in primary care. Four pillars supported the foundation of this paradigm: new diagnostic criteria, measures of the severity of illness, articulation of a biomedical framework, and a better understanding of the clinical epidemiology of emotional disorders in primary care. These pillars supported a platform for national educational campaigns in the United States and the United Kingdom. In both countries, however, leaders in psychiatry and general medicine realized that massive educational campaigns were simply the end of the beginning of the process of improving the quality of care for depression in primary care. In the following chapter, we review the extensive research effort in health services aimed toward continuing this effort.

10

FROM HELPING THE DOCTOR TO FIXING THE SYSTEM

In the previous chapter, we described efforts to reinvent the treatment model for depression in primary care that were largely driven by psychiatry. Having invented this new model, the psychiatry leadership confronted the enormous challenge of putting the new model into practice. To put the model into practice, medical educators and opinion leaders had to change the practice behaviors of primary-care physicians. Traditional methods to instruct practicing physicians in the new state of the art included articles in prominent journals or local lectures delivered by eminent teaching physicians. The DART and Defeat Depression campaigns are examples of this type of effort.

As this chapter demonstrates, changing primary-care practice is much more difficult than simply providing continuing medical education for physicians. Educating physicians about the new model is a necessary step, but not sufficient in itself to change practice. The primary-care leadership and other policy makers demanded evidence that the new model actually helped patients before they encouraged generalist physicians to adopt it. Perhaps most important, the new challenges of the primary-care practice environment (e.g., longitudinal care of chronic conditions) presented barriers to implementing the new recommendations for treatment of depression.

Disseminating the New Paradigm in Primary Care

Just after psychiatry recovered from the negative criticism about benzodiazepines and was beginning its new educational campaigns, the publication of *Listening to Prozac* ushered the new treatment paradigm into the 1990s (Kramer 1993). This book, and other similar publications, captured society's recurrent concerns about the effectiveness and proper boundaries of psychiatry and psychopharmacology. In 1993, the Agency for Health Care Policy and Research published new practice guidelines for treating depression in primary care (Depression Guideline Panel 1993). These guidelines were consistent with the message of the DART campaign, and the effort marked an awakening of the primary-care sector's interest in contributing to policy in this area: In fact, three of the guideline panel members were primary-care clinicians. Furthermore, the whole notion of "treatment guidelines," which physicians would have found distasteful only a decade earlier, was now the cutting edge of quality improvement. In the United Kingdom, general practice was attempting to incorporate not only quality-improvement practices but also the fundamental changes in practice precipitated by fund holding and the new Patient Charter described in Chapter 5. Health-services research sought to change provider behavior concerning the care of depression in primary care within this context.

There are multiple ways to view the educational strategies that the mental health leadership employed. Recall that the basic goals of these programs on both sides of the Atlantic were to educate primary-care physicians about how to recognize and manage depression and to educate the public about depression and the availability of treatment. These goals reflect the data demonstrating that most patients with mental illness do not seek care, that those who do seek care consult a primary-care physician, and that primary-care physicians often fail to provide state-of-the-art treatment. These goals also adopted the assumption that the current diagnosis and treatment choices developed in specialty psychiatry could and should be applied in primary care. Finally, the education strategy followed a story line that was well known to primary-care physicians through previous strategies implemented for hypertension, cholesterol, diabetes, and various cancers. Taken together, the efforts to change providers' behaviors in the care of depression passed through three stages.

The first stage, which began in the mid-1970s and extended into the 1990s, explored various strategies to improve providers' awareness and recognition of depression. These strategies relied on traditional modes of continuing medical education and attempts to improve attitudes. The second stage, which began in the late 1980s and continued through the 1990s, coupled diagnostic aids (patient-screening questionnaires to help identify potentially treatable depressive syndromes) with explicit treatment guidelines. The third stage, which began in the 1990s and continues today, coupled diagnostic aids with specific guidelines and with additional health-system or human resources to facilitate treatment (Callahan 2001). We describe the research exploring the effectiveness of each of these three stages.

Improving the Primary-Care Physician's Diagnostic Acumen

During World War II, military psychiatrists screened inductees for personality disorders, substance abuse, and mental disorders using self-administered questionnaires. Not only did these questionnaires prove to be an efficient mechanism to identify soldiers at risk for poor performance in the military, they also highlighted the prevalence of hidden or latent disorders. As described in previous chapters, numerous studies in the postwar period had reported epidemiological data on the prevalence of psychiatric morbidity in primary care and in community-based populations. By the 1970s, scientists were beginning to describe the prevalence of specific psychiatric disorders in primary-care settings using simple questionnaires. By the mid-1980s, the Epidemiologic Catchment Area study had reported the prevalence of specific psychiatric disorders in the community using a telephone survey. These efforts to identify patients with mental illness from large populations of adults produced screening tests for mental illnesses, including emotional disorders. Researchers wondered whether these questionnaires could help doctors detect mental illness among primary-care patients.

In 1976, *Lancet* published one of the earliest studies to address the effectiveness of providing primary-care physicians with the results of psychiatric screening scales. A. Johnston and David Goldberg (1976) completed a controlled trial testing the effect of providing General Health Questionnaire (GHQ) scores to primary-care physicians. Notably, the GHQ is not a depression-specific screening instrument; instead, it taps a broader range of physical and psychiatric distress symptoms than depression-specific instruments do. The generalist physicians' initial examination (without access to GHQ scores) resulted in a diagnosis of "conspicuous psychiatric illness" in 32% of their patients. In reviewing the GHQ scores, the authors reported that an additional 11.5% of patients had "hidden psychiatric morbidity." The investigators followed three groups of patients: *(1)* those with conspicuous psychiatric illness, *(2)* those with hidden illness whose GHQ scores the investigators did not reveal, and *(3)* those with hidden illness whose GHQ scores they provided to the doctor.

At 12-month follow-up, those patients with revealed psychiatric morbidity who suffered from a severe disturbance showed greater improvement in their GHQ scores. Outcomes among patients with milder disorders did not differ between the study groups. This study provided the first evidence that information support to primary-care physicians might improve both the process and outcomes of care. The study had multiple methodological shortcomings, however. Subsequent studies providing feedback on the GHQ to primary-care physicians failed to replicate this early study's findings (Hoeper et al. 1984; Shapiro et al. 1987).

Many investigators in this period tacitly assumed that primary-care physicians know their patients well and that treatment opinions offered by third parties are irrelevant. At the time, doctors would have considered "treatment guidelines" tantamount to "cookbook medicine." Yet a number of studies during the 1970s began to cast doubt not only on primary-care physicians' ability to diagnose and treat depression but also on the integrity of their long-term relationships with their patients. In other words, the problems of mental health care in primary care included underrecognition, undertreatment, and unfamiliarity between the doctor and patient. In a study published in the *British Journal of Psychiatry*, Johnson (1974) reported that 40% of depressed patients in a general practice in the United Kingdom felt that they were "not known" or "hardly known" to their family doctor. Other studies at this time, in both the United Kingdom and the United States, began to describe the low levels of detection and treatment of depression in primary-care settings in more detail (Callahan et al. 1996). Primary-care physicians' poor clinical performance opened the door for greater oversight and mechanization of their clinical practice. Thus, intervention strategies began to increase in sophistication, intrusiveness, and complexity. Investigators coupled greater informational support with reports of scores on psychiatric screening scales and treatment advice.

Linn and Yager (1980), reporting in the *Journal of Medical Education*, coupled feedback of depression screening questionnaires with a specific request that physicians give an explicit opinion about the patient's mood. The scientists designed this request to sensitize the physician to the presence of a potential mood disorder and their presumed responsibility in addressing the problem. The authors reported that screening and offering feedback of scores improved the physician's likelihood of making a notation about depression in the patient's medical record, but the intervention had no demonstrable effect on treatment rates. In addition, sensitization alone (not coupled with patients' scores on a depression screening scale) had little influence on the process of care. The scientists did not design the study to identify specific emotional disorders, and there was no objective measure of patient outcomes. There was a growing cadre of researchers examining the effectiveness of various forms of informational support to care for primary-care patients with emotional disorders.

In 1983, Zung and King (1983) provided the results of a study that was the first to report the beneficial effect of depression screening. The researchers screened 499 patients attending a general medicine clinic using a depression screening scale and formal diagnostic criteria. They randomized half of the patients meeting the criteria for depression to treatment with alprozolam (a benzodiazepine) and half to a control group. Patients in the control group received the "usual care" of their primary-care physician, which may or may not have included the diagnosis and treatment of depression. The investigators reported that 66% of subjects receiving the intervention improved in four weeks, compared with only 35% of the control group. Notably, the investigators, not the general practitioners, determined and monitored the treatments. The primacy of the primary-care physician in diagnosing and treating his patient because he or she "knew the patient the best" was beginning to erode. The researchers limited the study to a single practice, and they assessed outcomes only after four weeks, so this study had important limitations. The study does not provide evidence regarding the ability of screening questionnaires to improve the clinical performance of primary-care physicians. To make the results even more difficult to judge, the investigators chose benzodiazepines as their first-line treatment. The authors commented that outcomes with alprazolam were "comparable to the results in treating depression in a psychiatric practice using antidepressants." This provides another example of the treatment controversy regarding the use of benzodiazepines for primary-care patients with depression as discussed in earlier chapters.

In the period around 1990, three studies published in the United States evaluated the effect of providing patients' scores on screening instruments on primary-care physicians' practice patterns. In the first study, physicians provided the GHQ scores were more likely to diagnose depression than the control physicians were, but there was no difference in the likelihood of diagnosis for other psychiatric conditions (Rand et al. 1988). The second study, by K. Magruder-Habib and colleagues (1990) at Duke University Medical Center, provided primary-care physicians with their patients' depression-specific screening scale scores. In the intervention group, physicians recognized depression in their patients and initiated treatment for them more often. The study demonstrated that investigators could use the feedback from these scales to change primary-care providers' behaviors. The authors did not measure whether these changes affected patient outcomes.

The third study provided primary-care physicians with their patients' GHQ scores but coupled these data with specific feedback regarding their patients' desire for evaluation and treatment (Brody et al. 1990). Commentators had previously suggested that one reason so few patients presented their mental health concerns to primary-care physicians was their assumption that these problems were not in their physician's purview. Thus, extending an explicit invitation to discuss these problems and offering specific information about the primary-care physician's interest in providing treatment might improve treatment rates. The investigators showed some differences in care, and patients in the intervention group reported greater satisfaction with the mental health counseling they received. The study enrolled relatively few patients, did not identify specific psychiatric diagnoses, and did not report patient outcomes using standardized instruments, however.

One can begin to see how these studies progressed from continuing medical education intervention to facilitating recognition and diagnosis to involving the patient in requesting mental health care. Unfortunately, the changes in physician and patient behaviors achieved in these studies were modest and of unclear value. Primary-care physicians, their leaders, and those with fiscal responsibility for primary-care practices were increasingly demanding evidence of the cost-effectiveness of the screening programs. These demands began in earnest by the mid-1970s and gained in authority and acceptability throughout the 1990s. Thus, activists calling for routine screening for depression in primary care met with the same demands required of screening programs for colon cancer, breast cancer, and heart disease.

In 1990, the University of California–San Francisco and the National Institute of Mental Health convened a symposium to consider the case for routine screening for affective disorders in primary care (Attkisson and Zich 1990). Douglas Kamerow, then director of clinical preventive services at the Office of Disease Prevention and Health Promotion, was one of the speakers charged with reviewing the evidence. He concluded:

Although many of the necessary criteria for adopting a screening test for depression are satisfied, all of them are not. Depression is a common, important disorder, seen frequently in primary care, and there is no question that the use of currently available questionnaires will result in more cases being identified. Gaps exist, however, in demonstrating that early intervention in primary care patients with depression makes a difference and in rigorously documenting that the use of screening questionnaires can change patient outcome. (Quoted in Attkisson and Zich 1990)

Some have suggested that if researchers had applied as many resources to evaluating screening for mental disorders as they applied to test screening for cancer or heart disease, more answers would be available today (Attkisson and Zich 1990).

Demonstrating the Applicability of the New Paradigm in Primary Care

In 1991, the journal *General Hospital Psychiatry* began a new section entitled "Psychiatry and Primary Care." The editors established the special section having recognized that "most patients with mental illness are seen exclusively in primary care medicine" (Katon 1991). The editor of the new section was Wayne J. Katon from the University of Washington School of Medicine, and the inaugural paper in this series was by Herbert C. Schulberg at the University of Pittsburgh School of Medicine. Both of these investigators, and their colleagues at their respective medical schools, would prove to be among the most frequent contributors to the new field of psychiatry and primary care throughout the following decade. Schulberg and colleagues (1991) summarized the conundrum in which this new field found itself in the early 1990s:

Primary care physicians are being urged to provide patients experiencing a major depression treatments validated with psychiatric patients. The propriety of transferring clinical technologies from one care-giving sector to another is questionable, however, as it has little scientific support. . . . The course and outcome of primary care depressions are unclear and the evidence supporting treatment efficacy is sparse, selective, and below contemporary scientific standards. If the state of knowledge is to be advanced, researchers should design clinical trials capable of determining which treatments are effective with which depressed ambulatory medical patients. In so doing, investigators will be required to bridge what NIMH Director Judd has described as "the formidable gap between the comparatively pristine world of a clinical trial and the hurly-burly ambience of the service program operations" in which primary care research typically is conducted. Not surprisingly, few investigators have been inclined or able to bridge this gap.

An extensive literature described the incidence and prevalence of depressive disorders in the community, primary care, and hospital populations (Blacker and Clare 1987; Katon and Schulberg 1992). Campaigns such as the DART and Defeat Depression efforts were promoting treatment guidelines culled from the specialty psychiatry sector. At the same time, data emanating from primary-care settings hinted that these guidelines could not be clearly applied, and experts questioned the value of screening for depression. Even the experts could not produce data regarding which patients with emotional symptoms in primary care should receive which treatments. Also, these experts knew little about how to improve primary-care physicians' and their patients' adherence to recommended treatment. Furthermore, the poor clinician performance in achieving the recommended standard of care for depression was not limited to the primary-care sector in the 1980s. At least two large studies in the specialty psychiatry sector also demonstrated poor acceptance and application of these standards by community psychiatrists (Keller et al. 1986; Goethe et al. 1988).

Leaders in academic psychiatry were lamenting both the gap between knowledge and practice and the limited applicability of extant research to day-to-day clinical practice (Keller and Lavori 1988; Eisenberg 1992). Writing in the *New England Journal of Medicine* in 1992, Eisenberg commented:

What can be done to improve the care of medical patients with psychosocial distress? The answer does not lie in referral to mental health specialists; there are simply too few, and most of them are clustered in cities. Any realistic hope of change must rest on improving the quality of care in the general medical sector. For this, no single solution will suffice. There is a pressing need to increase knowledge of, and change attitudes toward, psychiatric disorders; help generalists improve their interviewing skills; develop a range of practical therapeutic options; and reshape reimbursement schedules. We cannot assume that training schemes will work simply because they are intuitively sensible. Rather, each potential intervention must be tightly coupled to an evaluation.

The energetic campaigns to improve the care of depression in primary care led by the psychiatric leadership in both countries did not fully consider the complex world of primary care. This complexity included competing disease priorities, the uncertain transferability of psychiatric lessons, difficult socioeconomic problems, discordant mental health care reimbursement, and the role of the patient. In the early 1990s, the experts were still sending an ambiguous message to primary-care physicians about treating depression.

The leadership in both psychiatry and general medicine began to realize that the effort to improve patient outcomes would have to move beyond interventions that relied solely on informational support to primary-care physicians. Not only were issues regarding the effectiveness of education and screening unclear, but the validity of the DSM-III diagnostic criteria in primary-care patients was uncertain, and the efficacy of the available antidepressant medications was questionable. Thus, in the early 1990s, researchers studying depression in primary care had to take a step backward and reevaluate the assumption that what worked in the specialty psychiatry setting among selective patients was equally applicable to the typical primary care patient. Schulberg and colleagues (1995) addressed this question in a large study funded by the National Institute of Mental Health in 1991.

In this study, the investigators randomized 283 patients with uncomplicated major depressive disorder to treatment with nortriptyline, interpersonal psychotherapy, or usual care (Schulberg et al. 1995, 1996). Usual-care patients received the typical care provided in a primary-care environment, which may or may not have included specific treatment for depression, depending on the individual physicians' decisions. Primary-care physicians and the research staff co-managed patients in the two intervention groups. The research team provided physicians, patients and staff with substantial encouragement and advice in order to facilitate adherence to the study protocol. Despite the resources afforded to both the intervention physicians and the patients, only one in three of the intervention patients completed a full course of therapy. Among those completing treatment, approximately 70% of intervention patients, compared with 20% of usual-care patients, recovered at eight months. These rates of response were comparable to those achieved in psychiatry. Notably, the authors published the study's results in a primary-care journal rather than a specialty psychiatry journal, even though most of the prior literature in this field had been published in psychiatry journals. Subsequent follow-up of these patients indicated that those who had completed a full course of therapy had improved overall functioning, as well as improvement in their depressive symptoms (Coulehan et al. 1997).

The study by Schulberg and colleagues raised as many questions as it answered. For example: *(1)* Was treatment only efficacious among patients meeting the research study's selective criteria? *(2)* Was treatment only effective if the intervention included the additional resources of pharmacotherapists and psychotherapists? *(3)* How should the larger group of patients with depressive symptoms not meeting the criteria for major depressive disorders be treated? *(4)* Why did two-thirds of the patients who agreed to participate in a research study and who received substantial additional health-care resources afforded by the clinical trial fail to complete the recommended course of treatment? *(5)* Could doctors duplicate these results in a typical primary-care practice with the typical primary-care patient with depression?

While the Schulberg study was being conducted, some developments in primary care and depression limited the study's relevance. For example, fluoxetine (Prozac) became one of the largest-selling drugs in the United States and precipitated yet another a backlash against the medicalization of social problems (Kramer 1993). The Agency for Health Care Policy and Research published new treatment guidelines for depression in primary care (Depression Guideline Panel 1993), scientists proposed new screening tools such as the PRIME-MD (Spitzer et al. 1994), and experts revised the diagnostic criteria for mental illness to be used in primary care (deGruy and Pincus 1996). Other scientists debated both the efficacy and specificity of antidepressant medications (Greenberg et al. 1992; Song et al. 1993), and researchers produced a growing body of evidence identifying depression as a chronic and recurring condition. Regardless, Schulberg and his colleagues demonstrated that, given adequate resources, doctors could effectively treat at least some primary-care patients with depression by applying the specialty psychiatry treatment paradigm.

Implementing the New Paradigm in Primary Care

Given evidence that the treatment model helped primary-care patients when it was delivered in the context of a research study, the next challenge was to help primary-care physicians organize their practices in such a way that they could implement the new depression-care model. Researchers distinguish between the value of the treatment under research conditions (efficacy) and the value of the treatment when provided in a real-world practice (effectiveness). Many factors in the real world of clinical practice may negate the potential value of a treatment. Examples of this include physicians prescribing the treatment incorrectly, patients not taking the medications, or patients' other medical conditions interfering with the treatment. Thus, researchers set out to study innovative strategies to get the right treatment into the right patient in the primary-care environment.

W. Katon and colleagues (1995) conducted a randomized clinical trial published in the *Journal of the American Medical Association* that compared the effectiveness of a multifaceted intervention in patients with depression in primary care with the effectiveness of usual care. The study team enrolled 217 primary-care patients, recognized as depressed by their primary-care physicians. Of these patients, 91 met criteria for major depression and 126 were diagnosed with minor depression; all of them agreed to treatment with an antidepressant medication. Intervention patients received more intense and frequent visits with their primary-care physicians and with a psychiatrist in the first six weeks after initiating the medication. Patients also received ongoing encouragement and surveillance to facilitate adherence to the medication, including education using videotapes and written materials. Patients in the control group received the usual care of their primary-care physicians.

Among the patients with major depression, the intervention group had greater adherence than the usual-care controls to adequate dosage and duration of antidepressant medication for three months or more. These patients were more likely to rate the quality of the care they received as good to excellent, and they were more likely to rate the antidepressant medications as helpful. Intervention patients with major depression were also more likely to report that their depressive symptoms had improved. Among patients with minor depression, the intervention group also had greater adherence, but there were no differences in depressive symptoms compared with the usual-care group. Notably, clinical outcomes of minor depressive disorders were good for both groups of patients, and the authors suggested that "usual care" for minor depressive disorders was more effective than previously appreciated.

The study by Katon and colleagues again found that, among a selected group of patients, strict adherence to recommended treatment guidelines improved patient outcomes. The study suggested that these same guidelines are not very applicable to patients who do not meet the criteria for major depressive disorders and showed that doctors needed substantial resources to ensure patient adherence to recommended levels of care. When doctors and patient do not achieve these recommended levels of treatment, clinical outcomes are worse. Unfortunately, this research team reported in follow-up studies that the intensive physician education had no lasting effects on physicians' practice patterns (Lin et al. 1997), depression-specific outcomes (Lin et al. 1999), disability, or health-related quality of life (Simon et al. 1998; Revicki et al. 1998). Prior commentators had suggested that improved treatment of depression might result in a decrease in total health-care costs (a cost-offset effect) by reducing depressed patients' use of general medical services. The University of Washington team did not show a medical cost-offset effect in its studies (Von Korff et al. 1998).

This finding can be explained by the changing definition of depression. Until about 20 years ago, the Kraepelinian view that depression was an episodic disease was popular. Between episodes, depressed patients were supposed to recover all at once and regain psychosocial competence. Views have since changed, and many now view depressive illness as an ongoing process punctuated by periods of clinical visibility. Clinical invisibility does not necessarily mean psychosocial competence, however. Depressed patients often disappear from the specialist's room but continue consuming mental health services elsewhere.

In the United Kingdom, two influential studies published in the mid-1990s added to the debate about the appropriate scope and quality of general practitioners' services. In 1994, researchers in Edinburgh completed a randomized trial "to compare the clinical efficacy, patient satisfaction, and cost of three specialist treatments for depressive illness with routine care by general practitioners"

(Scott et al. 1994). The study enrolled 121 patients who met the diagnostic criteria for major depression from 14 primary-care practices. The study team randomized patients to treatment with an antidepressant prescribed by a psychiatrist, cognitive behavioral therapy from a clinical psychologist, counseling by a social worker, or routine care by a general practitioner. The investigators documented marked improvement in depressive symptoms in all treatment groups over four months. There was only a marginal clinical advantage of the specialist treatments over routine general practitioner care, and these therapies "involved at least four times as much therapist contact and cost at least twice as much as routine general practitioner care." The authors questioned whether the additional cost of specialist care would be worth the minimal clinical advantages demonstrated in the study.

In the other U.K. study, researchers at Oxford University conducted a clinical trial to test the feasibility and effectiveness of a brief psychological treatment delivered in the primary care setting for major depression (Mynors-Wallis et al. 1995). The researchers randomized patients to a brief problem-solving treatment, an antidepressant medication, or a placebo and followed them for three months using the Hamilton Depression Rating Scale. The problem-solving therapy required six sessions and about three and one-half hours to deliver. Patients who received the problem-solving treatment and patients receiving medication showed significant improvement compared with the placebo group. There was no difference in outcomes between the groups treated with antidepressants and the group treated with the brief psychological treatment. The authors concluded that this brief form of psychological therapy was both feasible and effective for treating major depression in primary-care settings. Although this was a relatively small study, it provided evidence that psychological treatments were effective and that doctors could tailor them to fit in with the day-to-day practice of general medicine.

In the last quarter of the twentieth century, more than a dozen clinical trials assessed how enhanced information support could improve the recognition and treatment of depression in primary care (Callahan et al. 1996; Callahan 2001). These studies increasingly combined information support with more direct support of clinical decision making for individual patients. Information support might include access to treatment guidelines and even data on which patients in the practice have depressive symptoms. Support of clinical decision making would include more patient-specific data on how to treat an individual patient and how the patient responded to treatment over time. Researchers then combined this decision support with greater resources (e.g., nurse care managers) to help implement standard treatments.

Eventually, scientists began to explore more complex features of the primary-care health-care system. The science of improving the care of patients with depression had moved away from passively providing educational materials to understanding that changing provider behaviors required changing the system of primary care. The science had moved away from a strategy of admonishing primary-care physicians to a strategy of altering their practice environment in a manner that helped them do the right thing.

In 1998, Schulberg, Katon, and others reviewed the reports of randomized controlled trials in primary-care settings published between 1992 and 1998. These investigators concluded the available data supported the view that "both antidepressant pharmacotherapy and time-limited depression-targeted psycho-therapies are efficacious when transferred from psychiatric to primary care settings" (Schulberg et al. 1998). They also suggested that

improving treatment of depression in primary care requires properly organized treatment programs, regular patient follow-up, monitoring of treatment adherence, and a prominent role for the mental health specialist as educator, consultant, and clinician for the more severely ill. Future research should focus on how guidelines are best implemented in routine practice, since conventional dissemination strategies have little impact.

The 1990s began with an enthusiasm among the mental health leadership that continuing medical education targeted to primary-care physicians would result in the rapid transformation of primary-care practice patterns for depression. How to improve general practitioners' standard of care for their patients with depression proved to be much more complex than expected, however. Like other chronic conditions, such as diabetes or heart disease, adopting the newer methods of screening, diagnosis, treatment, and long-term management of depression required both physician education and fundamental changes in the primary-care practice environment. In large part, these changes called for substantial cost outlays for additional human resources and capital expenditures to transform primary care from an acute-care to a chronic-care delivery system. The problem was particularly complex because primary care had never even successfully incorporated an acute-care model for mental disorders:

There is now an explosion of knowledge about mental disorders, and it at last becomes possible to discern the outlines of a model for mental disorders which takes account of findings in both social psychiatry and molecular biology. However, we have not made corresponding progress in refining the administrative and architectural requirements for meeting the needs of the mentally ill, and in most countries of the world services for the mentally ill survive on the crumbs left from the banquet of general health care. (Goldberg and Huxley 1992)

Wagner and colleagues (1996) described the extent of the changes needed to improve the care of chronic conditions in primary-care settings. For any chronic condition, patient education and physician informational support are necessary but not sufficient for precipitating improvement. Treatment guidelines based on evidence of effectiveness and the availability of treatment are simply a place of departure. Both physicians and patients also need access to resources to improve communication, collaboration, and self-care. Medical informatics (using computerized medical records to support physician decision making) offered the promise of supporting physicians' information needs and providing a vehicle for decision support (McDonald et al. 1992, 1999). In the 1990s, physicians were growing more accustomed to the types of systems redesign that they might have viewed as intrusive in the past. For example, it is no longer unusual for a physician to receive a reminder from a computer, a pharmacist, or a nurse care manager to consider a change in treatment for a given patient. In fact, the presence of computerized medical records and a team approach to care are now considered evidence of quality care.

Augmenting the System of Care

One of the more effective sets of strategies tested across several studies and reported in the early twenty-first century consisted of interventions that combined information support with both a care manager and longitudinal tracking of patient outcomes. A care manager is typically a non-physician health-care professional whose primary role is to assure that patients with depression receive guideline-level treatment. We describe four such studies here. Each study used a slightly different approach to redesigning the primary-care practice environment in order to help generalist physicians adhere to treatment guidelines. Each study provides a slightly different menu of additional resources. Thus, each of these four systems approaches to improving quality would be associated with additional costs to the health-care system.

The first such study (Wells et al. 2000) tested a quality-improvement program in a randomized clinical trial conducted in 46 primary-care clinics associated with six different managed-care organizations. The investigators randomized 1356 patients with major depressive disorder to one of three types of clinics: *(a)* usual care, *(b)* a quality-improvement program including a local nurse to improve medication adherence, or *(c)* the quality-improvement program plus access to psychotherapists. The quality-improvement program included an institutional commitment, training of local experts to provide professional and patient education, and a screening program to identify potential patients. At six months, about 60% of the depressed patients in the quality-improvement groups had improved, compared with 50% of the controls.

In the second study, investigators tested the effectiveness of usual care with feedback alone or feedback coupled with *(a)* treatment recommendations, *(b)* practice support from a care manager, or *(c)* longitudinal tracking using regular telephone contact (Simon et al. 2000). Feedback in this study consisted of information on current antidepressant drug use, rather than feedback regarding the severity of the patient's depressive symptoms. The researchers identified as potential subjects those whose doctors had recently prescribed them an antidepressant, based on computerized pharmacy records. Feedback of information support and passive access to practice guidelines did not affect either the process or the outcomes of care. In the group also receiving care management, patients were more likely to receive an adequate dose of the antidepressant and were more likely to experience fewer depressive symptoms.

Katzelnick and colleagues (2000) took a slightly different approach in which they identified primary-care patients (enrolled in three different HMOs) with high health-care use. Among the 1465 patients so identified, investigators enrolled 407 who had evidence of depression. They then randomized patients to either usual care or a depression-management program that included professional and patient education, coordination of care using telephone contacts, and pharmacotherapy managed by the primary-care physician. Patients in the intervention group were more likely to be treated with antidepressants and had significantly improved depression scores and general health status compared with the usual-care patients. At six months, about 56% of patients in the care-management group had improved, compared to 40% in the usual-care group.

In the fourth study, Unützer and colleagues (2002) reported the findings of a multi-site clinical trial testing a collaborative-care model in primary care. A depression clinical specialist (typically a nurse) led the collaborative care, working in collaboration with a team of providers, including the primary-care physician and a consultant geriatric psychiatrist. Much of the care, however, was coordinated by the depression clinical specialist, using an algorithm that defined a stepped-care approach. In the stepped-care approach, patients begin treatment with a relatively simple treatment plan. If they do not respond, the providers gradually increase the intensity of the treatment. The study involved 18 primary care clinics from eight health-care organizations in five states and enrolled 1801 older adults with late-life depression. Many of these patients had multiple co-morbid chronic medical conditions treated with multiple medications. For up to 12 months, intervention patients had access to a depression care manager who received supervision from a psychiatrist and a primary-care expert. The care manager offered education, care management, and support of antidepressant management by the patient's primary-care physician or problem-solving treatment in primary care. At 12 months, 45% of intervention patients had a 50% or greater reduction in depressive symptoms compared to 19% of usual-care participants. Intervention subjects also experienced less functional impairment and greater quality of life than participants assigned to usual care.

These studies focusing on improving resources and restructuring the health-care system provided excellent evidence that doctors could successfully treat the depression of medically complex primary-care patients. They also continued to expose the limited effectiveness of the care that patients in primary care usually received. Furthermore, many of these findings suggested the need for a fundamental redesign of primary care and a newer team approach to care that did not necessarily place the primary-care physician in command. Although these system-level interventions proved to be effective, critics noted the unanswered questions about cost-effectiveness and whether health-care systems could afford to provide the additional resources needed for the care of depression. In addition, experts began to shift attention away from the primary-care physicians and toward the role of patients in seeking help, accepting treatment, and taking an active role in their care.

Summary

By the 1980s, researchers understood that educational campaigns would not change provider or patient behaviors. These campaigns were more effective in articulating a framework to define a standard of care than in providing a method to change behaviors. Early interventions to change provider behaviors initially focused on efforts to improve their recognition of depressive symptoms and then addressed other methods to provide informational support. The goal was to help practitioners achieve guideline-level treatment because the intensity of treatment in primary care was often low. By the end of the twentieth century, these interventions evolved toward more complex strategies that coupled informational support and practice guidelines with increased human and physical resources. While many of these interventions have led to demonstrable improvements in the process and outcome of care, policy makers still grapple with how to pay for these additional resources. Given these findings, researchers have moved toward models of care that focus on prevention, patient lifestyle, and self-care. In the next chapter, we discuss the limitations of the current treatment model from the perspective of both individual patients and entire communities.

Part III

LESSONS LEARNED AND MOVING FORWARD

11

BOUNDARIES AND LIMITATIONS

In the first two parts of this book, we described the broad scope of social and scientific factors that are important in explaining the current treatment model for depression. This includes discoveries in psychiatry and psychopharmacology, as well as primary care and clinical epidemiology, and it includes social changes that experts often have viewed as external to medical care. We highlighted the fundamental role of primary care in treating people with emotional disorders and outlined the history of symptoms and treatments for emotional disorders in primary care. Around 1990, psychiatry offered a new treatment model for caring for people with depression, with a particular emphasis on care provided by generalist physicians. In this chapter, we discuss the limitations of that model.

Boundaries of Mental Health Care

Before discussing the limitations of the current treatment paradigm for depression in primary care, it is important to distinguish how the model is limited due to the boundaries imposed by cultural values. Cultural values dictate how far science can go in offering its potential remedies for various ills and how it should present and prioritize its findings. Though there are many such boundaries, ranging from human subject concerns in biomedical research to the acceptable adverse effects from treatments, we focus on debates at two macroscopic boundaries: First, the

mystery versus the machinery of the human mind; second, individual liberty versus social responsibility and conformity. While science and culture play important roles in these debates, we argue that these boundaries are more contentiously
debated for mental illness than they are for medical illness. The real issues, however, are that people debate the boundaries, and these boundaries change over
time.

On June 26, 1907, Oxford University bestowed honorary degrees of Doctor of
Letters on two writers. One, Rudyard Kipling, won the Nobel Prize for Literature
in 1907, the first English author to win the award. Born in India at the time of
British rule in the mid-nineteenth century, Kipling's writings often looked backward by celebrating Victorian England, Imperialism, and British patriotism. The
second writer honored that day with the pronouncement "most charming, most
facetious man, you who shake the borders of the whole universe by your inborn
merriment" (Rodney 1993) was an American. Mark Twain was not above irrever-
ence in his writings on England, and he turned the focus of American fiction away
from Europe and toward America. At the turn of the twentieth century, the United
States was gaining enough confidence in its own culture and history to begin to
both celebrate them in writing and to seek a course different from that of the
United Kingdom.

By the early nineteenth century, classical psychology, neuroanatomy, and
phrenology converged into what was to become the new science of neurophysiol-
ogy. This included a new language for describing nervous activity and the old tri-
partite division of the mind as suggested by Kant. After some debate, experts
applied both types of description to understanding madness. Schizophrenia and
paranoia were to become disturbances of thought; depression, mania, and anxiety
disturbances of emotions; and the personality disorders an aberration of the will.
During this first organicist period in the history of psychiatry, the semantic structure on which psychiatry grounded the mental disorders was surrendered in favor
of direct correlations between brain changes and overt complaints. Freudianism
can be considered as one reaction to such an important loss of meaning (Berrios
1988, 1996).

The language of emotional symptoms provided a shared social meaning, or an
explanation, for why the patient felt the way they did. In the past, patients,
providers, and societies had negotiated labels for emotional symptoms in a manner that embraced their origin. Treatments focused on symptoms rather than on
any notion of reversing the origin of the symptoms. The origin was typically a
stressor (both past and present) that resided in the environment and often outside
the purview of medical care. In the late twentieth century, psychiatry began to
suggest that the etiology of the emotional disorder could be found in biochemical
derangements in the brain. In other words, psychiatry advocated a mechanistic
explanation for why people felt happy or sad. To many patients, this explanation
summed up an individual as so many component parts—some working and others

not working. People and societies still struggle with the notion of "man as a machine." As is earlier centuries, participants frequently flavor these struggles with semantic arguments.

In 1906, a year before receiving his honorary degree at Oxford, Twain captured the man versus machine debate in his book *What Is Man*. He wrote the book as a debate between an old man and a young man, and the following excerpt summarizes their opposing views:

OLD MAN: There are gold men, and tin men, and copper men, and leaden men, and steel men, and so on—and each has the limitations of his nature, his heredities, his training and his environment. You can build engines out of each of these metals, and they will all perform, but you must not require the weak ones to do equal work with the strong ones. In each case, to get the best results, you must free the metal from its obstructing prejudicial ores by education—smelting, refining, and so forth.

YOUNG MAN: You have arrived at man now?

OLD MAN: Yes. Man the machine—man the impersonal engine. Whatsoever a man is, is due to his make, and to the influences brought to bear upon it by his heredities, his habitat, his associations. He is moved, directed, commanded, by exterior influences-solely. He originates nothing, not even a thought.

YOUNG MAN: Oh come! Where did I get my opinion that this which you are talking is all foolishness?

OLD MAN: It is a quite natural opinion—indeed, an inevitable opinion—but you did not create the materials out of which it is formed. They are odds and ends of thoughts, impressions, feelings, gathered unconsciously from a thousand books, a thousand conversations, and from streams of thought and feelings which have flowed down into your heart and brain out of the hearts and brains of centuries of ancestors. Personally you did not create even the smallest microscopic fragment of the materials out of which your opinion is made; and personally you cannot claim even the slender merit of putting the borrowed materials together. That was done automatically—by your mental machinery, in strict accordance with the law of that machinery's construction. And you not only did not make that machinery yourself, but you have not even any command over it.

Twain, who rarely shied away from controversy, delayed publishing the book for at least a decade, thus reflecting the controversial nature of this subject. When he finally did publish it, he did so privately and only produced 250 copies. Writing in *Science* magazine over 90 years after Mark Twain's treatise, Charles Nemeroff, a leading figure in pharmaceutical research, could pen such statements as "the mind, however, does not exist without the brain." He could do so without fear of public reprisal from his university, the state, or the church. Regarding the debate about the etiology of depression Nemeroff (1998) wrote:

Psychologists and neurobiologists sometimes debate whether ego-damaging experiences and self-deprecating thoughts or biological processes cause depression. The mind, however, does not exist without the brain. Considerable evidence indicates that regardless of the initial triggers, the final common pathways to depression involve biochemical changes in the brain.

While researchers and others have the intellectual freedom to consider the bio-chemical basis of emotions at the beginning of the twenty-first century, the same data do not necessarily convince society, at least not at the same speed. Thus, at present, there is a widening knowledge and communication gap between science and society. Pharmacotherapy for mental illness contributes to this gap in the same way as do genetically-modified foods, gene therapy, cloning, evolution theory, and the loss of privacy through technology. Scientists may produce knowledge, tech-nology, or strategies that society does not believe are ethical, safe, or affordable. This leads to arguments not about the quality of the science but the about the mer-its of applying the science. The scientists tend to get stuck on logical arguments about the potential good of their discovery and overlook society's fear about the potential harm. In the area of mental illness, the argument often involves the rela-tive importance given to man as the machine versus man as the spiritual being. No-tably, the fears about an overly mechanistic view of mental illness are not limited to nonscientists. Consider this thesis from a medical sociologist:

No matter how closely the internal electronics of a television set are examined they will never reveal an adequate understanding of the type and variety of programmes being shown; in the same way, an examination of the brain, no matter how detailed, can never succeed in explaining why someone has a certain thought, or holds a religious or political belief, or speaks a particular language. (Armstrong 1994)

In the realm of diagnosing and caring for emotional illness, psychiatry and primary-care leaders must negotiate with society about labels and how treatments are connected with these labels. If society views the real etiology of depression as a stressor in the environment (e.g., unemployment), then treatments that focus on medications will be poorly received by patients. Unfortunately, many environ-mental stressors may be outside the purview of primary care.

This leads us to the second cultural boundary—that is, the question of how hard medicine can push to change human behavior without infringing on individual rights. To what extent should society legislate against such high-risk behaviors as neglecting to wear seat belts and motorcycle helmets, smoking cigarettes, eating a poor diet, and excessive drinking of alcohol? For medical professionals, where is the boundary between education and coercion? If medical experts provide an indi-vidual with access to health information, should we accept a seemingly reckless decision such as riding a motorcycle without a helmet in the name of freedom of choice? Might high-risk activities for one person be safe for another? Where is the boundary between personal choice and addiction? Mark Twain, a lifelong cigar smoker, was already over 70 years old when he accepted his honorary degree at Oxford. At his 70th birthday celebration two years earlier, he is credited with the aphorism, "We can't reach old age by another man's road. My habits protect my life but they would assassinate you" (*New York Times*, 1905).

The issue of how responsible medicine and society at large should be in shaping or controlling individual behavior is a contentious problem that remains unresolved. This is a vexing problem for primary-care physicians because we entrust them with promoting healthy lifestyles. Public health experts in the United States listed tobacco, diet, activity patterns, and alcohol as the top contributors to mortality (McGinnis and Foege 1993), with firearms, sexual behavior, motor vehicle accidents, and drug abuse also in the list of top-10 contributors. Scientists identify these contributors as causing most chronic conditions, which accounted for 75% of U.S. health-care expenditures, or $659 billion, in 1990 (Hoffman et al. 1996). Thus, personal behavior becomes a societal problem when viewed through the lens of societal health-care expenditures and a limited national budget.

Some analysts point to this focus on the control of lifestyle behavior as a clear example of medicine overreaching its boundaries. Petr Skrabenek (1994), a physician researcher in the department of community health in Trinity College, Dublin, has been one of the more recent writers raising the alarm:

The pursuit of health is a symptom of unhealth. When this pursuit is no longer a personal yearning but part of a state ideology, healthism for short, it becomes a symptom of political sickness. Extreme versions of healthism provide a justification for racism, segregation, and eugenic control since "healthy" means patriotic, pure, while "unhealthy" equals foreign, polluted. In the weak version of healthism, as encountered in Western democracies, the state goes beyond education and information on matters of health and uses propaganda and various forms of coercion to establish norms of a "healthy lifestyle" for all. . . . The proclaimed aim of healthism is the "health of the nation" with an implicit promise of greater happiness for all. However, there is a world of difference between attempts to "maximise health" and those to "minimise suffering." As Karl Popper pointed out in "The Open Society and Its Enemies," all attempts to maximise the happiness of the people must lead to totalitarianism.

The boundary between normal fluctuations in emotional symptoms and major depressive disorder is constantly changing. The boundary between facilitating access to care and coercing patients to seek care is unclear. The boundary between encouraging a patient to adhere to a medication and pressuring him or her to comply with the recommended standard of care is ambiguous. The boundary between relieving the burden of emotional symptoms at a societal level and becoming an agent of repression in facilitating socially sanctioned inequities is cloudy. The boundary between treating mental illness and altering basic personality traits is controversial. Different cultures, societies, interest groups, physicians, and patients draw different lines between encouraging participation and coercing participation. What society might find acceptable for "encouraging" participation differs, depending on whether one is treating communicable diseases, preventing heart disease, or treating emotional symptoms.

The Challenge of Changing Behavior

In 1894, Mark Twain wrote that "habit is habit, and not to be flung out the window by any man, but coaxed downstairs one step at a time." An individual often must change behaviors to prevent, treat, or manage an illness, whether the illness is medical or mental. Some behaviors are so intractable that scientists have described them as hardwired into the human genome. Others are influenced by social norms, and thus people might be able to change. We place the challenge of changing behaviors as both a boundary and a limitation of the current model for treating depression. The patient's role in preventing and managing chronic conditions has been a slowly developing research area over the past 40 years. As applied to emotional disorders, increased patient participation implies enacting appropriate help-seeking behaviors, effectively communicating symptoms to the provider, participating in selecting among treatment choices, bearing the financial cost of care, and adhering to this plan of action for years.

Armstrong (1988) reviewed the historical origins of the interest in individuals' health and illness behaviors. He noted that society has transformed the early twentieth century concept of "health" as one side of a dichotomy into a concept of health as a continuum with unclear boundaries between health and illness. This transformation has important ramifications for patient expectations. Earlier in the twentieth century, according to Armstrong, the physician viewed disease as a pathologic lesion residing within an individual. This individual was a repository of a disease; while the physician dealt with this disease, the individual was more or less a passive observer. As the lessons of personal hygiene and lifestyle behaviors became increasingly understood, patients became more active participants in improving their health and in improving the overall conditions for health in their local environments. As the lessons of prevention became increasingly understood, patients became not just active participants but "self-practitioners." Doctors have transformed the former patient into an integral member of the health-care team.

Before World War II, doctors viewed patients as nonparticipants in accepting health care only if they failed to seek help for symptomatic disease. At the end of the twentieth century, nonparticipation also included failure to engage in behaviors that might prevent disease:

One of the effects of recruiting the patient as an integral component of health management was the change in the status and nature of "patient" identity. The boundary between healthy person and patient became problematic. In the past, we marked "coming under the doctor" as the transition from person status to patient status. In the new regime which made the patient both an object of medicine and a lay health practitioner, patienthood began to lose its old meaning. This shift was marked by extending patient status as everyone came under health surveillance as we recruited everyone to the medical enterprise. Post-war surveys of population morbidity and symptom prevalence confirmed that a rigid distinction between health and illness was meaningless; everyone had health problems, everyone was "at risk." Health care merely touched the tip of the morbidity iceberg. In addition, the now problematic boundary between person and patient was subjected to a close analysis in the new subject of "illness behavior." (Armstrong 1988)

However, this new conception of the patient as participant also has a dark side. Taken to its extreme, society can judge patients as responsible for their illnesses. Some experts argue that this dark side caused a shift in focus away from such social determinants of health as poverty, poor education, and stifled opportunities and toward a focus on individuals failing to protect their health:

The major effect was to lessen the concern with the role of social factors in health and illness and to place emphasis on individual psychological factors in health and illness. The focus moved away from the social environment: housing, work, income, and macro factors towards coping, stress, social support, health lifestyles, and activities located in the individual. The locus for change which might improve the public health [has] clearly shifted to the person and away from society. (Research Unit in Health and Behavioral Change, University of Edinburgh 1989)

The double-edged sword of increasing patient participation versus increasing social control of individual lifestyles comes with risks: "The public health of continuous surveillance is at once both liberating and repressive, a beam of enlightenment held in the grip of a spectre of total social control" (Armstrong 1988). Mental illness accentuates these issues. The boundaries between illness, health, better than healthy, and social control constitute one of the main themes in Kramer's (1993) *Listening to Prozac.*

Unfortunately, it has proved extraordinarily difficult to change lifestyle behaviors. Public health officials bombard people in the United States and the United Kingdom with information on exercise, diet, smoking cessation, blood pressure control, seat belts, cancer screening, alcohol and drug abuse, and a plethora of other behaviors. Efforts in primary care related to emotional disorders include attempts to educate patients about the symptoms of depression, the availability of treatment in primary care, and the importance of adhering to medications. Recent nationwide examples include such educational programs as the "Depression-Awareness, Recognition, and Treatment" in the United States and "Defeat Depression" in the United Kingdom. Although the impact of these efforts typically goes undiscovered, when researchers do measure these campaigns' outcomes, the effect is minimal. Individuals rarely change behaviors simply as a result of having communicated data about health risks that may apply to them. The Research Unit in Health and Behavioral Change at the University of Edinburgh summarized this phenomenon:

The recognition that health-related activities are intimately bound to existential and structural systems has been belatedly acknowledged in the new term "health promotion." Indeed, the recent promotion of health promotion seems to be based, at least in part, on the tacit acknowledgement of the failure of conventional health education to demonstrate any significant direct links between its various activities and campaigns and changes in health-related behavior. It seems that an understanding of how behavior changes in the context of everyday activities and adaptations would provide a more enlightening and practical basis for planned interventions. (Research Unit in Health and Behavioral Change, University of Edinburgh 1989)

In attempting to change patient behaviors related to emotional disorders, researchers confronted the same barriers that had proved to be insurmountable for other public health problems. Subtle efforts to change behaviors are often ineffective, and strong-arm tactics can be both ineffective and counterproductive. While the biomedical model that viewed mental illness as a discrete disease helped bring more science and credibility to the study of psychiatry, it may have devalued the social determinants of mental illness and the importance of help-seeking behavior and self-care. Kickbusch (1998) summarized this dilemma:

Here lies the challenge to develop new types of research on health behavior based on an ecological model of health that sees the individual as an integral part of a social group and acknowledges the biological as well as the nonbiological component of health. In such a perspective, health is multi-dimensional phenomenon; the interaction between individuals and their social and physical environments is understood as integrated and holistic.

Interestingly, few people disagree with assessments such as this one. Unfortunately, translating these recommendations into a research agenda, a clinical practice, a system of health care, or a public policy is extraordinarily difficult. So difficult that such a translation appears to be out of reach in the near future for both the United States and the United Kingdom.

Limitations of the Current Treatment Model

There are three important limitations of the current treatment paradigm. First, even under ideal conditions, 25% to 30% of primary-care patients with major depression fail to respond to the current treatment model. Specialty psychiatry researchers, clinicians, and policy makers all recognize this limitation (Lebowitz et al. 1997). Whether one views this limitation as the cup three-quarters full or one-quarter empty, we still have a treatment paradigm that, even in the best of hands, has room for significant improvement. This alone is reason to argue for a continued critical reappraisal of the existing treatment model. Second, primary-care patients with symptoms that do not meet the criteria for major depressive disorder get better with nonspecific treatments provided in the usual care of primary care. Yet, many of these patients are mistakenly treated with antidepressant medications because the demarcation between these symptoms and the syndrome of depression can be difficult to identify. This is particularly true in primary care, where the patient's other chronic medical conditions might produce some of these symptoms. Third, many patients in the community with depression do not seek care for their symptoms. In the following sections, we discuss these latter two limitations in more detail because they represent the hidden limitations of the current model.

During the 1990s, evidence began to accumulate that many of the depressions supposedly "missed" by primary-care practitioners had a more indolent course than those that were recognized and treated. Goldberg and colleagues (1998) completed a study to describe the outcomes of patients with depressive illness whom doctors had diagnosed compared with patients the doctors failed to diagnose. The researchers collected data from 15 cities throughout the world, including cities in the United States and the United Kingdom. They sorted patients into four groups: those treated with an antidepressant; those treated with a sedative, those diagnosed but not treated, and those with unrecognized depression.

Patients treated with antidepressants or sedatives had a similar severity of depression and similar prior histories of depression; patients who did not receive drugs had less severe depressive illness. Given the dissemination of the new treatment model discussed in Chapter 10, the researchers' findings were surprising. They found no relation between drug selection and diagnosis. For example, doctors prescribed antidepressants for patients receiving a research diagnosis of depression about as frequently as for anxiety or somatoform disorders. The same was true for other drugs.

Patients whom doctors chose not to treat had a better course over the following year. Among the patients doctors had treated, outcomes were similar among the three groups. Two-thirds of patients treated with drugs remained symptomatic at the end of the year. Patient adherence to recommended dose and duration of the drug was poor. The researchers commented:

Patients not given drugs had milder illnesses but did significantly better than those receiving drugs, both in terms of symptoms lost and their diagnostic status. Unrecognized depressions were less severe than recognized depressions, and had a similar course over the year. Patients receiving antidepressants were better in terms of overall symptoms and suicidal thoughts than those treated with sedatives at three months, but this advantage does not persist. Depression emerges as a chronic disorder at one-year follow-up—about 60% of those treated with drugs, and 50% of the milder depressions, still meet criteria for caseness. The study does not support the view that failure to recognize depression has serious adverse consequences, but, in view of the poor prognosis of depression, measures to improve compliance with treatment would appear to be indicated. (Goldberg et al. 1998)

The current treatment paradigm still leaves the primary-care physician with considerable uncertainty regarding who needs treatment, what treatment they need, and how to achieve adherence to the treatment. Epidemiological data suggesting that those with milder forms of depression are at higher risk for developing more severe forms of depression leave the primary-care physician with considerable uncertainty regarding the boundaries between risk reduction, prevention, and treatment.

In describing the third limitation, that many people with depression never seek treatment, we integrate the first two limitations as well. Through this integration, we provide a conceptual model for why the burden of depression remains so high in the United States and the United Kingdom, despite important improvements in our understanding and treatment of depression. Doctors do not diagnose all patients with depression who present themselves for care, and they do not treat all patients they diagnose. At the same time, patients whom doctors diagnose do not necessarily accept or adhere to treatment when doctors prescribe it, and patients treated by doctors for depression do not always get better.

Epidemiological data demonstrate that a large group of people with emotional problems relies on self-care or care outside the formal health-care system to deal with its problems. We refer to this pathway as "informal health care." By informal care and self-care, we mean measures as diverse as counseling from a religious authority, enrolling in a meditation class, herbal therapy, or extricating oneself from a crisis, among myriad other possible interventions. Finally, some people eschew formal care, informal care, and specific measures for self-care altogether. This may be because they do not view themselves as ill or because they view the hazards of seeking care as greater than the hazards of the disease. Figure 11–1 depicts the three possible routes that a person might pursue when addressing emotional symptoms.

The model starts on the far-left side in the middle box, with the reservoir of individuals with symptoms. These individuals have three alternatives: (A) seek informal care or self-care, (B) attempt no specific care measures, or (C) seek care in primary care. The figure does not depict a pathway to specialty care because of the limited number of people traversing that pathway relative to the other three pathways. Some patients, however, will find a path directly to psychiatry. Each of the three alternatives is bi-directional because if individuals are not satisfied with one alternative and remain symptomatic, they may consider a different alternative. Also, the bi-directional arrows imply that certain circumstances may facilitate or inhibit travel through those alternative pathways. (We discuss those circumstances later in this section.) For simplicity, the figure does not depict a pathway for individuals who choose both pathways A (informal care) and C (primary care) at the same time.

Because we know a great deal about the process of care in primary care, the figure shows the major steps in care as separate decisions, each of which is bi-directional. There may be important subcomponents of care in informal health care also, but we don't know enough about informal health care to delineate them. Each of the three pathways (A, B, and C) has a documented rate of achieving remission of symptoms. We denote these rates as follows: pathway X (recovery through informal care), Y (spontaneous recovery), and Z (recovery through formal care). Finally, among those individuals who achieve remission and become asymptomatic, there are definable rates of recurrence among those with prior

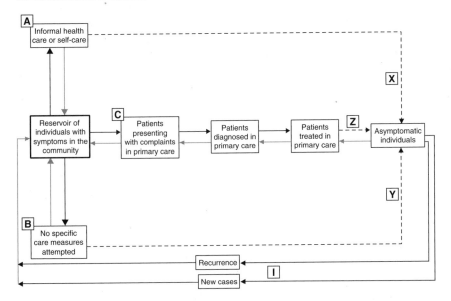

FIGURE 11–1. Three care options for people with emotional symptoms (A, informal care: B, no care; C, primary health care) and the corresponding remission rates associated with these options (X, informal care, Y, no care, Z, primary health care). I denotes the incident rate of depression among asymptomatic individuals.

episodes and incident cases among those with no prior episodes. These rates are denoted as I on the figure.

Cultural factors affect which of the three paths an individual chooses. Also, among those choosing formal health care, differences in the health-care systems could lead to significant differences in the rates of diagnosis and treatment. If people with depression choose alternatives A (informal care) and C (no care) more often than alternative C (formal care), the primary health-care system's design becomes less important. Also, if pathways X (recovery through informal care) and Y (spontaneous recovery) achieve remission rates approaching pathway Z (recovery through formal care), the primary-care system's effectiveness becomes less important. Finally, if the sum of pathways X, Y, and Z (total recovery rate by any means) is greater than pathway I (the incidence and recurrence of disease), then the prevalence of depression in the community will decrease.

In Figure 11–2, we depict factors that might lead individuals to seek and receive effective care in primary care, as well as factors that might reduce the incidence of disease. The curved arrows and the factors listed next to them depict factors that move people in the direction of the straight arrow to which the curved arrow is attached. Thus, this figure shows factors that move people into the formal health-care pathway. Cultural factors, such as accepting a medical model for treatment, perceptions of the degree of disability, and social stigma, have impor-

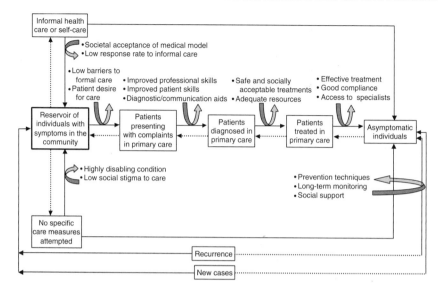

FIGURE 11-2. Factors that facilitate people choosing care for emotional symptoms in the formal health care system. Thin solid arrows depict successful movement through the formal health care system and a decrease in the number of persons with emotional symptoms. Thin dotted arrows depict unsuccessful movement through the formal health-care pathway and an increase in the number of persons with emotional symptoms. Curved thick arrows depict the factors that facilitate successful movement through the different stages of the formal health-care system.

tant effects on the number of patients with emotional illness choosing each pathway. The magnitude of these effects translates to greater or lesser emphasis on the effectiveness of care within the primary health-care system. As Figure 11–2 shows, the effectiveness of the primary-care system is imperative because each factor suggests that most individuals would seek care in primary care. The effectiveness of primary care becomes paramount in this situation, and the prevalence of depression in the community directly reflects the quality of primary care.

Figures 11–1 and 11–2 are relevant to many other symptomatic conditions or illnesses, but the route that individuals choose will differ depending on the condition, the availability and effectiveness of treatment, and the cultural milieu. Consider, for example, the difference in people's rates of choosing the three alternative pathways if they were experiencing the common cold, as compared to influenza, bacterial pneumonia, or a fractured leg. Sometimes, there can be a dramatic change in the preferred pathway over time because of medical discovery and changes in social stigmata, such as in the case of men with erectile dysfunction. The advent of an effective medication results in more people seeking treatment, while simultaneously removing some of the condition's former stigma by re-framing it as a biomedical rather than a psychosocial disease.

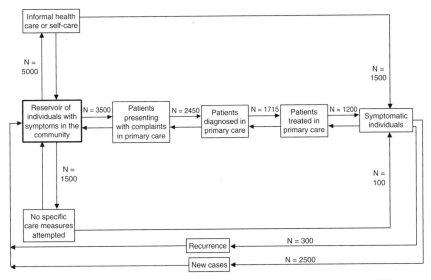

Population of 100,000 patients with 10% prevalence of depressive disorder and yearly incidence of 2.5%

FIGURE 11–3. Depiction of a steady state reservoir of people with emotional symptoms despite availability of effective treatment. This model includes a population of 100,000 people and assumes a 10% prevalence of depressive disorder and a yearly incidence of 2.5%. Treatment and recovery rates for the three routes of care are taken from reports in the literature.

Using the diagram in Figure 11–2 and data from the epidemiological studies described in this book, we can show how the prevalence of depression could reach a steady state. We also can show how factors outside of primary care modulate its potential impact on the burden of depression in the community. Figure 11–3 depicts a population of 100,000 individuals with a prevalence of depression of 10% and a yearly incidence of 2.5%. The model assumes that 50% of patients with depression will choose informal care or self-care treatment, 35% will choose to seek care in primary care, and 15% will not attempt specific treatment. We assume a placebo response rate of at least 30% for those choosing informal care (pathway A). This does not necessarily mean that the proffered treatments in informal care are placebos. Because we do not know the effectiveness of most of these informal treatments, we assign them at minimum a placebo response rate. The model assumes no treatment response for no care (alternative B). Based on results regarding usual care in primary care in the United Kingdom and the United States, the model assigns a response rate of 34% for those choosing formal care in primary care (alternative C). We calculated this figure by assuming that doctors will diagnose 70% of patients who present with depression, they will treat 70% of those diagnosed, and 70% of those treated will have their symptoms resolved.

Using these assumptions based on solid data, we find that structural differences in primary care in the United States and the United Kingdom have had only a modest influence on the prevalence of depression in the community. Also, the prevalence of depression remains steady over time, despite the availability of effective treatments because the rate of cure equals the rate of new or recurrent illness. Using the available epidemiological data, this model indicates that the current treatment model will not produce a substantive decline in the prevalence of depression because it places too great an emphasis on the minority of people who follow the pathway of formal care.

Field Studies of Boundaries and Limitations

Obviously, this model's assumptions are debatable. Some readers might argue for a much higher response rate in the informal care and no specific care pathways, while others might argue for lower rates. However, we have presented a wealth of data within the formal health-care system regarding response rates in research studies (efficacy) compared with response rates in specialty psychiatry settings or primary care (effectiveness). We also can support the formal care response rates presented in Figure 11–3 with data from individual studies. However, we cannot point to studies that test the full model. The model explains a wide variety of findings from the extant literature in both clinical epidemiology and health-service research on emotional disorders in primary care. It also explains the substantial existing reservoir of disabling emotional disorders in the United States and the United Kingdom, despite advances in the treatment paradigm. Most important, it demonstrates how important both patients' help-seeking behavior and self-care behavior are on the effectiveness of the current treatment paradigm for depression in primary care. We next present two field studies that provide additional support for the conceptualization of the strengths and weaknesses of the current treatment paradigm, as depicted in the figures in this chapter.

In 1972, Barry Gurland in the United States and John Copeland in the United Kingdom embarked on a study to examine differences in the prevalence of dementia, depression, and disability in the two countries. They also sought to explore the effects of sociocultural differences on the prevalence and outcomes of these problems (Gurland et al. 1983). The investigators assembled a random sample of 445 older adults in New York and 396 older adults in London. The participants completed a battery of tests, including structured measures of symptom severity and formal diagnostic interviews. The researchers reinterviewed participants one year later.

Gurland and Copeland had hypothesized that the national health-care system in the United Kingdom would provide a greater safety net for older adults than the U.S. health-care system would. Contrary to their expectations, however, the team found no difference in the rates of depression between the two cities (13% in New York and 12.4% in London). Because social stressors were more severe in New

York and social services were less available, the investigators had anticipated that rates would be lower in London. Rates of physical illness, disability, and dependence were similar in the two cities, as were perceptions of the social stressors. Unfortunately, although subjects in both cities had access to ambulatory health care, patients with depression were unlikely to receive treatment specific to their illness. Although formal health-care services provided in the home were more available in London, informal services provided by the family were more available in New York. Thus, the sum of formal and informal health care was similar in both cities. The authors concluded:

The overarching impression gained from the cross-national comparison discussed here is that the health and social problems of the elderly in the two cities are more similar than dissimilar but the health and social services have cross-nationally differing styles and emphasis. There is no clear evidence in this study that the management of depression, dementia, or disability in the community is dramatically better in one or the other city though there is some edge in favor of the formal primary care and home care services in London and specialist care and the family role in New York.

In the mid-1980s, investigators at the Netherlands Institute of Primary Health Care conducted a study in their country, which has a health-care system with a design somewhere between that of the systems in the United States and the United Kingdom. The researchers had hoped to learn more about the gap between the observed need for mental health care according to psychiatric criteria and individuals' actual demand for help (Verhaak 1995). In the Netherlands's health system at the time of the study, about 60% of the population was publicly insured, but general practitioners served as gatekeepers for both privately and publicly insured patients. The investigators sought to address:

[the] discrepancy between mental disorder, as defined by psychiatrists and the patients' demands, deduced from requests for help. . . . · Either a lot of people suffer in terms of psychiatric standards, but do not share these standards, or a lot of people suffer but do not seek help, or a lot of people suffer but they are not recognized as suffering. (Verhaak 1995)

The study built on Goldberg's findings describing the pathways to mental health care, but the Dutch investigators were specifically interested in the operating features of the filters to care that Goldberg had described. In this study, the researchers recorded all physician visits among a population of 335,000 patients visiting 103 Dutch general practitioners during a three-month period. The investigators then selected a random sample of 16,000 of these patients to interview. Their goal was to assess mental disorders in the community, help-seeking behaviors related to these disorders, the complaints that patients presented to the general practitioners, and the general practitioners' response to these complaints.

The Dutch study collected data on reported mental distress and troublesome situations, as well as GHQ scores. The investigators found that 37.6% of the population had experienced a psycho-social problem indicative of mental distress in the previous two weeks. Women, older respondents, homemakers, and the unemployed had higher rates of symptoms than other groups. Over 50% of the respondents reported a troublesome situation such as "bad prospects for the future," difficult family relationships, or financial problems. About 9% of males and 16% of females scored above the threshold on the GHQ. This threshold identified subjects with significant symptoms of depression as defined by research criteria. The authors summarized that "many people experience problem situations, quite a lot of them have had feelings of mental distress, and a relative minority score above the threshold on the GHQ." Notably, more than half of those who reported feelings of mental distress had not consulted their general practitioner. Furthermore, even among those experiencing all three conditions—mental distress, a troublesome problem situation, and a high GHQ score—only about one-third discussed their problems with their general practitioner. The investigators suggested that many of these patients "find other solutions than medical care for their mental disorder. . . . Our data show that there are no serious limitations to the access to care." Patients with high GHQ scores were the most likely to present their psychiatric complaints to a general practitioner and were the most likely to receive a psychiatric diagnosis. The most common forms of treatment were psychotropic drugs and nonspecific counseling. The authors concluded that "a lot of people suffer according to psychiatric standards but their suffering is labeled differently, they seek different solutions, and their doctors approve of it" (Verhaak 1995).

While many of the studies discussed earlier in this book provided data for the individual components of the model depicted in Figure 11–3, these two field studies provide support for the overall model. This model explains why the burden of depression remains stable in the face of new and effective treatments. Perhaps most important, this model indicates that improvements in how primary-care physicians apply the current model will have only a limited influence on the community's health. This is true because so few people who might benefit from medical care actually seek this care. Also, the content, approach, and effectiveness of the current medical treatment model do not appear to attract this large reservoir of untreated depressed persons into the formal health-care system. We find little evidence, at least, that the current model is any more efficient in bringing people into the medical-care system than prior approaches were. Thus, while the current treatment model in the best of hands may help as many as two-thirds of individuals who meet specific characteristics, its limitations are such that the burden of depression in the community remains unchanged.

The Case of Suicide

When evaluating the effectiveness of public-health interventions, policy makers often seek hard evidence of the intervention's overall effectiveness. In the case of hypertension, for example, researchers reported that better control of hypertension results in a reduction in deaths from heart attack, stroke, and all-cause mortality. This is important for two reasons. First, it is conceptually possible that controlling blood pressure could have had no impact on these outcomes, or perhaps it decreased deaths from heart attack but increased death from strokes. Second, it is conceptually possible that control of hypertension might decrease death from stroke and heart attack but increase death from cancer. The recent controversy about estrogen replacement in women provides an example of a treatment that appears to improve symptoms and intermediate outcomes but increases the likelihood of death from other causes.

Because most patients who commit suicide suffer from depression, one might hypothesize that effective treatments for depression would reduce the overall rate of suicide at the community level. Thus, suicide provides another benchmark that demonstrates the boundaries and limitations of the current treatment model. Over the past century, suicide rates among older adults have been consistently higher than any other age group. Despite the media attention focused on suicide among adolescents and younger adults, people over age 65 are more likely to commit suicide (Diekstra 1995). The highest rates of suicide are found among Caucasian men over 70. In nearly all countries, there are important differences in rates and trends among the different race–gender groups. Suicide rates reported for older adults are consistently much higher in the United States than in the United Kingdom. Among adult men aged 75 and older, the suicide rate in the United States is 56.6 per 100,000 population, as compared to 21.6 per 100,000 in the United Kingdom (Gulbinat 1995). In contrast, rates of depression in the two countries are about the same. In general, U.S. suicide rates for older adults have increased over the past few decades, whereas they have decreased in the United Kingdom (Murphy and Wetzel 1980; Gulbinat 1995; Kennedy 1996).

Scientists link suicide in older adults to an extensive list of physical, emotional, and social problems (Kennedy 1996). Cultural factors have a role, as suggested by the magnitude of variation in rates of suicide across different countries and across different age cohorts within countries (Diekstra 1995). Because prevention is the only means of reducing death from suicide, early efforts have focused on identifying risk factors or risk profiles that might identify patients likely to contemplate suicide. The most consistent modifiable risk factor found in these studies has been depression. To date, however, no study has demonstrated reductions in overall suicide rates due to more effective treatment of depressive illness.

Even the effectiveness of suicide-prevention centers, which have existed in most large cities in the United States and United Kingdom since the 1950s, has been difficult to demonstrate (Dew et al. 1987). Also, older adults make only 4% of calls to suicide hotlines, even though they have the highest suicide rates (Kennedy 1996). As Kennedy explained: "Despite major advances in the health and economic well-being of older Americans, in the 1980s late-life suicide became more prevalent than at any time in the previous 50 years." In the 1990s, suicide rates among some groups of older adults have slightly declined. Both psychiatric and sociocultural factors are important in understanding suicide in late life.

Beginning in the 1970s, epidemiological research indicated that primary-care physicians had seen most older adults who committed suicide shortly before their death (Murphy and Wetzel 1980; Diekstra and van Egmond 1989; Frierson 1991; Conwell et al. 1991). Thus, public health officials viewed primary care as a potential site for suicide interventions, especially to reduce the rate of suicide in late life. Notably, most studies have found that even though primary-care doctors had seen these patients recently, the patients rarely raised concern about depression or suicide. Indeed, public-opinion polls found that "more than three quarters had not talked about suicide before the attempt" and only "13% had sought any form of help before attempting suicide" (Kennedy 1996). Unfortunately, there is a lack of research that would help primary-care physicians identify and treat suicidality in older adults. Except for a paucity of studies attempting to design screening instruments to improve recognition, there have been no randomized trials of suicide prevention in primary care. The National Institutes of Mental Health funded the first attempts to investigate primary-care-based interventions in 1999.

Fluctuations in suicide rates both within countries and between countries over the past 50 years have led to speculation that restricting access to lethal means of suicide might be an important intervention to reduce rates (Lester 1995). Brown (1979) reported that a reduction in the carbon monoxide content of domestic gas supplies in the 1970s was a major determinant in reducing England's suicide rates. Indeed, Brown found that attempted suicides actually had increased during this time. However, decreased access to highly lethal means of suicide, coupled with improved technology in the treatment of poisonings, led to an overall reduction in suicide deaths. In the United States, public health officials link suicide rates to rates of handgun ownership, as well as the carbon monoxide content of automobile exhaust (Lester 1995). There is some evidence that if individuals' preferred method of suicide is not available, then they will not necessarily substitute another means (Lester 1995). If this is true, then reducing access to lethal methods could be an effective way to prevent suicide in older adults. The existing data suggest that these efforts are at least as important as changes in primary care.

While some experts recommend decreasing access to lethal means of suicide, others seek to increase older adults' access to the means for a physically and emotionally comfortable suicide. One of the most controversial issues in geriatrics at the beginning of the twenty-first century is the debate over physician-assisted suicide and the boundaries between euthanasia and the right to die (Quill et al. 1992). While some experts see mental illness in those who think of suicide, others see self-determination. This sympathy toward patient autonomy is especially strong in decision making regarding end-of-life concerns among older adults. The

hope of providing for a peaceful death results in an ongoing tension between perceptions of ageism and neglect on the one hand and paternalism and the overzeal-
ous medicalization of death on the other hand.

Much debate on these issues will occur in both the United States and the
United Kingdom before these conflicts are resolved. This controversy demonstrates the enormous sociocultural influence over definitions of mental health and
the boundaries of health care. It also shows how societal characteristics can mar-
ginalize the effectiveness of the formal health-care system, regardless of its basic
design, focus on primary care, or attempts at universal access.

Has the Stigma of Mental Illness Changed?

Our argument about the limitations of the current treatment paradigm relies on
such evidence as the burden of depression in the community, including the overall prevalence of symptoms, syndromes, and suicide. Our argument also considers the established, modest effectiveness of the available treatments. However,
one other potentially very important benefit of the current model is its ability to
reduce the stigma associated with mental illness. In other words, the current
model not only provides safe treatment options but also reduces the stigma associated with seeking treatment. While we already have suggested that the literature
does not support the notion that people are more likely to seek treatment, those
who do seek treatment might be less stigmatized by the health-care system and
the community. Even in the absence of increased efficacy, the current model
could be beneficial to sufferers because it provides a biomedical model of illness
that removes the stigma and fear of mental illness.

As one avenue to examine society's acceptance of mental illness, we consider
the treatment of mental health issues over the past few decades of presidential
politics in the United States. Take, for example, *Newsweek*. On July 24, 1972, the
cover showed Democratic presidential candidate George McGovern and vice-
presidential candidate Thomas Eagleton with their clasped hands raised in a symbol of unity as they embarked on their quest for the White House. Two weeks
later, the brooding visage of Eagleton filled the cover, and one week after that
image, the cover featured the replacement Democratic vice-presidential candidate
Sargent Shriver. The Democrats had dropped Eagleton from the ticket. The courts
had not convicted him of a misdemeanor, treason, or infidelity. Rather, the press
discovered that doctors had hospitalized Eagleton three times (1960, 1964, and
1966) for nervous exhaustion. During these hospitalizations, he had twice undergone electroconvulsive therapy. Eagleton admitted to the hospitalizations but also
produced statements from his doctors that he had been well for some time.

Newsweek published a poll showing that 76.7% of 1015 eligible voters felt that
Eagleton's medical record would not affect their vote, but only 53.7% felt that Ea-

gleton was qualified to be vice president. Of those who said he was unqualified to be vice president, 50% said he was unqualified because of his psychiatric history, and 33.5% said he was unqualified because he had not come forward about his history of psychiatric illness. *Newsweek* also published a "poll" suggesting that patients who had been treated for depression did not think Eagleton should be a vice-presidential candidate.

In August 1988, *Newsweek* reported that Democratic presidential candidate Michael S. Dukakis "was accused of having received psychiatric treatment," and the *Washington Times* had published a story with the interesting headline, "Dukakis Psychiatric Rumor Denied" (Randolph 1988). When reporters asked President Ronald Reagan to comment on the rumors, he joked that he wasn't going to pick on an invalid. At issue was whether Dukakis had suffered from depression following the death of his brother, who had a history of mental illness. Dukakis eventually released the full details of his medical records to dispel the rumors. Treatment for mental illness, regardless of whether it was successful or remote, was a political liability, at least until 1988.

One reason to believe that societal attitudes toward mental illness are gradually improving is the positive public response afforded to Vice President Al Gore's wife, Tipper Gore. Mrs. Gore announced her own struggles with depression and was able to facilitate greater awareness of mental illness without damaging her husband's political standing. Mrs. Gore helped organize the first White House Conference on Mental Health in June 1999. Her efforts also were cited as part of the stimulus for the "First Surgeon General's Report on Mental Health." The U.S. Department of Health and Human Services announced the report in a press release on its web page in December 1999:

The report proposes broad courses of action that will improve the quality of mental health in the nation. These courses of action include continuing to build the science base, overcoming stigma, improving public awareness of effective treatment, ensuring the supply of mental health services and providers, ensuring delivery of state-of-the-art treatments, tailoring treatment to age, gender, race and culture, facilitating entry into treatment and reducing financial barriers to treatment.

Ironically, in the same month that the surgeon general's report was released, an Associated Press article reported that Republican presidential candidate John Mc-Cain was forced to release details of his medical history. The story reported that "documents were released in part to counter what McCain aides have called a 'whisper campaign' engineered by GOP presidential rivals challenging his mental fitness" (Fournier and Neergaard, 1999). America viewed John McCain as a national hero for his physical scars as a prisoner of war, but his emotional scars signified weakness. Such episodes raise doubts about how far the field has progressed in removing or reducing the stigma of mental illness.

Other evidence for the lingering stigma of mental illness includes disparity in third-party reimbursement for mental health care compared to medical care. Patients cite evidence of discrimination from employers, insurers, and others when their problems are labeled as psychiatric. Patients often ask their doctors to label their mental illness or mental illness treatments as due to medical illness. Doctors often comply and not infrequently knowingly miscode depression as chronic fatigue, insomnia, or some other physical symptom. There is evidence of progress, but there is also a clear need for further improvement.

Summary

There is considerable professional and societal ambiguity about the proper boundaries of primary care, psychiatry, and medicine. For most of the twentieth century, primary-care physicians were concerned only with patients presenting to the formal health-care system. Furthermore, even among patients presenting for care, primary care historically has been concerned with the patient's demands that they communicated as symptoms. Primary care had not been concerned with asymptomatic illness or unvoiced needs to be discovered by the physician or defined by public health officials. Public health, preventive health, behavioral medicine, and psychiatry increasingly have suggested that primary care's gaze must include people who do not seek formal care. We sometimes define people without symptoms as ill, and we ask these people to become their own practitioners. Because cultural factors influence concepts of illness, disease, and help-seeking behaviors, the relative importance of alternative pathways to care varies by disease and by nation. Because these factors vary by the perceived availability of treatment, there can be large changes in the volume of people choosing the different pathways without any change in the background prevalence of the condition.

The current treatment paradigm for depression in primary care has important boundaries and limitations. A wealth of clinical epidemiological data and studies of current patterns of clinical practice, help-seeking behaviors, and self-care demonstrate how depression can remain a major public health problem despite a half-century of discoveries related to diagnosis and treatment. Depression rates and the social stigma associated with depression have improved in some respects and remained unchanged in others. The main focus of the psychiatry treatment paradigm over the past half-century has been care for patients with severe mental illness. Psychiatry can claim enormous advances in the treatment of these patients. The main focus in primary care, however, has been the care of patients with emotional symptoms. Primary care has less evidence of significant advances in the care of these patients. From a public health perspective, the burden of depression in the community remains substantial. Only in the past decade or so have psychiatry and primary care begun to collaborate on a treatment model for the milder forms of depression seen in primary care.

We have presented a help-seeking and treatment model that suggests future efforts to reduce the overall societal burden of emotional disorders would have to move well beyond the formal health-care system. The boundaries that individuals and societies place on concepts of mental health constrain the latitude of such movement. In Chapter 12, we discuss how science and society might negotiate these boundaries in a manner that decreases the burden of depression in the community.

12

DEAD RECKONING AND MOVING FORWARD

We cannot move forward with purpose if we do not understand where we are and how we got here. Many wonderful histories of psychiatry are available, including studies of nosology, diagnosis, and treatment, as well as biographies of many of the great minds in psychiatry and psychology. Our goal has been much different. We have sought to provide a history of treatment for depression. Such a history cannot be told without weaving in the threads of primary-care doctors and patients because the formal care of emotional disorders takes place largely in primary care. Our goal has been to use this broader perspective as a navigational aid to determine where we are, how we got here, and where we need to go. With a better understanding of this history, we can avoid repeating some mistakes and repeatedly relearning lessons that are already well documented. Sir Geoffrey Vickers (1984), an expert in human behavior and complex systems, decried this problem in government's attempts to define the goals of public health:

It is a fact strange beyond comprehension that the whole corpus of human knowledge is re-learned at least three times each century; and this becomes even stranger when we remember that what is re-learned is not only the technological skills and knowledge which serve our common needs, but also the political and cultural ways of thinking and feeling and acting which determine what we shall conceive our common needs to be, and how we should pursue them.

Where Are We?

Founded in 1675, the Greenwich Observatory is located on the high ground in Greenwich Park, several miles downstream from London on the River Thames. Designed by Christopher Wren, the purpose of the observatory was not to learn about the origins of the universe but to catalog the positions of the moon and stars as a method to aid navigation at sea. The astronomers' goal was to develop a celestial-based method to determine longitude at sea. Although mariners had long before developed a mechanism to establish their latitude, the only method to determine just how far east or west one had sailed was by "dead reckoning" (Sobel 1996). Dead reckoning, derived from the phrase "deduced reckoning," is a method for approximating one's position based on a ship's course and speed. Navigators established the course with a compass and estimated speed by throwing an object overboard and reckoning the speed with which the ship moved away from the floating object. Closer to shore or on a river, a landmark might serve as a point of reference to gauge speed. They then plotted a series of vectors on a map. Estimating the influence of wind, current, and myriad other factors, the navigators hoped to determine the ship's position on the open sea.

In the twenty-first century, both distant and local observers can identify the position of nearly any object anywhere in the world within a few meters using satellite technology and the Global Positioning System. In a similar way, through the efforts of expert panels and systematic reviews, it is fairly straightforward to identify the medical profession's current position regarding the diagnosis and treatment of depression in primary care. Looking backward to how we got here and looking forward to where we are going are much more difficult tasks. This book has provided a historical account of the development of the current treatment paradigm for emotional disorders in primary care. To re-create this story, we relied on dead reckoning by using historical data to identify the point of departure and then to estimate the magnitude and direction of the influential vectors of the past 50 to 75 years. Understanding the entire range of factors that have acted on the course and direction of our current treatment paradigm is fundamental to developing a reasonable explanation of how we got here.

Failing to map and understand this history contributes to the notion that changes in the diagnosis and treatment of emotional disorders in the second half of the twenty-first century were planned, systematic, revolutionary, radical, and unprecedented. Thus, analysts using a more narrow perspective have pointed to the historical development of the present treatment model as a rational accretion of scientific discoveries, which suggests that scientists built each new finding on an earlier, reified foundation of facts. This linear progression of science, interrupted only by the paradigmatic shifts wrought by revolutionary discoveries, has provided a neat and convenient framework for how medical science decides about effective treatments for patients. Ample evidence, however, has shown that serendipity, social constructs, political forces, and societal changes have had at least as much influence on our treatment models as have either science or technology (Bloor 1991; Aronowitz 1998).

Understanding where we are and how we got here is fundamental to any attempt to forecast where we are going or where we might want to go. A broader perspective becomes particularly important when trying to understand the day-to-day behaviors of primary-care physicians, patients, and nonpatients. Therefore, this book has touched on aspects of the history of psychiatry as well as on primary care, health-care policy, therapeutic discovery, and important social influences. In identifying where we are, we must recognize that the public conceptions of mental illness do not necessarily move as quickly or as logically as professional conceptions do.

Returning to Recurring Themes

Five themes recur throughout the development of our current treatment model for depression in primary care. These themes represent the basic arguments of this text, and the preceding chapters presented the evidence for these arguments.

> 1. Trends set in motion by the Second World War II continue to influence Anglo-American health care. These trends include changes in demography, health-care resources, health-care systems, therapeutics, biomedical research funding, and mental health care policy.

For many practitioners born after World War II, the ancestry of much current medical practice is shrouded in a veil that overemphasizes the role of science. Understandably, these practitioners believe that clinical categories and the language constructed for describing them have solid, "scientific" credentials. Hence, in their view, all that society now needs are larger and more costly neurobiological research projects to identify the brain basis of all mental disorders. With the data presented in this book, we suggest that psychiatry in general and the treatment of the emotional disorders in particular may benefit more from low-cost historical, social, and conceptual research than from extensive brain research. These areas remain understudied in ascertaining the nature and structure of mental disorders.

The practical exigencies of war stimulated much innovative science and serendipitous discovery. The research infrastructure and scientific credibility of psychiatry, in particular, enjoyed a transformation during World War II, and this credibility boost provided the psychiatry leadership with the confidence to extend the reach of psychiatry into more complex areas of social debate. Although not explicitly stated previously, the stories retold in this book demonstrate that World War IIsignificantly affected the lives of future leaders in medicine, many of whom were on very different career trajectories before the war. The war did not just change the direction of their careers; it helped shape how people thought about disease, therapeutics, research design, the sociology of disease, and science's role in tackling the nations' problems. This is part of the story of how medicine arrived at its current position, and it reveals the typically unplanned nature of scientific developments.

2. The history of our current treatment paradigm for depression is no older than about one generation. The constant flux of social constructs and the malleable interpretation of scientific facts have resulted in a plasticity of help-seeking behaviors and clinical practice styles for emotional disorders. The treatment model has changed and should continue to change.

For at least two reasons, it is important for primary-care physicians, among others, to recognize the fluctuating landscape of care for depression. The most obvious reason is that the recommendations for caring for any given illness will always be in flux, and medical science does not determine this flux in isolation. Moreover, patients may have different perspectives from those of their physicians, which may be a source of tension in the doctor–patient relationship. It is not possible for physicians to consider their patients' viewpoints if they cannot back away slightly from a biomedical model. As Armstrong (1994), a medical sociologist, explained:

The patient does not come to the doctor with the odd isolated symptom but with a comprehensive belief system which in its range and power rivals the biomedical scientific belief system of the doctor. Therefore, although on the surface the doctor–patient relationship might be categorized by common interests and a common goal, it can be seen to represent a meeting of two different "experts" each with their own explanations about the nature of illness, its causes, its prognosis, and its appropriate treatments.

To the extent that Armstrong's depiction is accurate, this represents an extraordinarily difficult environment in which to deliver primary care. Yet, Armstrong's sociological perspective is echoed in the sentiment of the primary-care leadership:

Most often, physician and patient meet on terrain that is neither of certainty nor of scientific ignorance, and the use of either large-scale, formal research studies or "point and shoot" therapy seems inappropriate. The art of medical care involves a continuing individualized search in which the physician tries to match incomplete scientific knowledge of disease and treatment with incomplete local knowledge about particular patients at particular times in their lives. (Berwick 1998)

There is reason to believe that "incomplete local knowledge about particular patients" is a growing problem because the physician–patient belief systems are continuing to diverge while expectations are increasing. This is occurring because society is not keeping pace with biomedical discoveries and the gap between the patient's and the physician's understanding of the biomedical model continues to widen. This explains a great deal of the public's dissatisfaction with medical care at the beginning of the twenty-first century. According to Kaufman (1993):

The upheavals brought about by the embrace of the scientific enterprise and the proliferation of innovative technological and pharmacological tools radically altered both physicians' and the public's notion of responsibility and possibility in medicine—and that transformation happened in one lifetime. The process of change itself and, more important, the ramifications of change for the tasks of medicine and for American society were unplanned and, with few exceptions, unexamined. In fact, medicine's metamorphosis was accidental, the result of meeting countless day-to-day challenges in patient care and clinical research with the tools, models, and practices of the biomedical sciences. Both the rapidity with which that transformation occurred and the fact that is was unpredictable, unanticipated, and not subject to scrutiny or evaluation have contributed to contemporary medicine's moral quandaries.

This conception may explain some of the disparities between the physician's medical knowledge and the patient's health behavior and compliance. It also may partly explain the explosion of interest in complementary or alternative medicine.

3. Definitions of health and illness are ephemeral, but the goals of health care, and the patients and physicians themselves, have remained more constant than popular lore suggests. Patients' help-seeking behaviors for emotional disorders and physicians' basic skills and comfort with these disorders have not changed substantively over the past half-century.

Research findings over the past 50 to 75 years have indicated that emotional problems have always been a prevalent complaint in primary care. They also suggest that most patients with these problems, when they decide to seek formal health care, seek care from primary-care physicians. Over the past century, primary-care physicians have rather consistently treated these complaints with a combination of counseling and symptomatic medications. These types of treatments have responded to a clear patient demand. The interaction of medical advances and social constructs has dramatically affected how patients and providers frame patients' symptoms. This framework affects both the potential patients' decisions to seek care and the providers' decisions regarding what care to dispense. Within a decade, enormous numbers of British and American citizens shifted from seeking care for their nerves and receiving treatment with benzodiazepines to seeking care for depression and receiving treatment with antidepressants. Writing in 1982, when benzodiazepine use was at its peak, Parish argued that

by their use of these drugs, doctors clearly define to patients a model for dealing with certain symptoms produced by unpleasant situations. Doctors' prescribing habits therefore influence patients' expectations which subsequently determine demands.

Doctors are not insulated from influence, both subtle and overt, whether it is from their patients or from science, pharmaceutical companies, or society.

4. Patients' needs and expectations and physicians' desires to provide health care are always at least slightly higher than the competence, capac-

ity, and resources of the available health-care system. While this mismatch may create a healthy tension that leads to quality improvement and ultimately better health, it also overshadows the improvements in health care, including mental health care, that have accrued over time.

Patients, health-care providers, and society at large all have growing expectations regarding health outcomes. Mark Twain was only four years old when his father died. He buried two of his daughters who died from infectious diseases, and one of his daughters was repeatedly hospitalized for extended stays in a mental facility. He also buried his wife. When Twain was born, life expectancy was less than 40 years; by the time he died in 1910 life expectancy was just over 50 years, and by the end of the twentieth century it was 75 years. At the turn of the nineteenth century, fewer than 50% of all children survived to age 65. At the turn of the twentieth century, 80% of children lived to age 65 and 30% lived to age 85 (Kramarow et al. 1999).

Whether these remarkable improvements are due to public health as opposed to biomedicine is not relevant to the current argument. The point is that longevity has increased over the past century, and many would argue that this reflects the community's improved health. Developments as diverse as safe anesthesia and pain control, heart transplants, treatments for osteoporosis, and an entire field of preventive medicine have made better health a real possibility for millions of people.

This enormous success does not quench society's appetite for even better solutions to health problems, however. Also, the listed health benefits are unevenly distributed in both the United States and the United Kingdom. Improvements in mortality have brought the gigantic problem of chronic disease, and technological improvements have ignited serious social arguments. Regardless, the care of severe mental illness is better today than it was in 1940, and the medical care delivered in primary care is safer and more effective than it was in 1940. In addition, the care of mild to moderate emotional disorders in primary care is at minimum safer than it was at that time.

Vickers (1984) suggested that "the history of public health might well be written as a record of successive redefinings of the unacceptable. " At one time, asylums for patients with severe mental illness were viewed as progress. Perhaps one day we will view nursing homes for older adults as warehouses for the aged and deem them unacceptable. There are many examples of health-care problems that used to be accepted as inevitable or at least tolerable that have become viewed as unacceptable in the twenty-first century. Vickers also noted that "the amount of effort which can plausibly be devoted to the health of the individual and the community increases with every scientific development, and will, I think, increase indefinitely." Many societies already face the prospect of limiting the amount of national resources that they can allocate to health care.

5. Science, society, and health care intersect in primary care. Most patients with depression seek and receive care from primary-care providers. Improving the care of patients with depression will depend on improvements in primary care. It will also depend on the outcome of debates about the reach of medical science into the lives of people who do not view themselves as requiring medical treatment.

Rates of depression across developed countries have not fallen because new pharmaceuticals have been discovered, whereas rates of infectious diseases have plummeted as antibiotic use and public health measures have increased. At the same time, rates of depression have not fallen as better understanding of prevention and multifaceted treatments have become available, whereas deaths due to heart attack and stroke have fallen. Some of this gap between discovery and outcomes may be due to gaps between knowledge and practice in primary care. We argue that this gap between what we know and what we do in primary care is only a small part of the problem. Reinventing depression will demand that we negotiate with the community about how mental illness is defined and how far medical care should reach into private lives.

A Leadership Role for Primary Care

Over much of the twentieth century, primary care has been a voracious receiver of new treatments, new care recommendations, new roles, and new responsibilities from patients, researchers, specialists, public health experts, and policy makers. As the place of first contact for patients seeking care for the full range of human conditions, primary care has been celebrated for its potential and vilified for its failures. In any given year over the past 50 years, one could go to the medical literature and find both a call for the rebirth of primary care and an obituary mourning its death. One also could go to the literature and find a whole series of human conditions for which primary care reportedly is failing the public trust.

Primary care is supposed to be the place for health education, prevention, timely treatment of acute conditions, and long-term management of chronic conditions, as well as where we prepare for a dignified death. Primary care is meant to address both emotional problems and physical problems and understand their relationship. Primary care should be equally prepared to care for victims of domestic violence and victims of the common cold. Nutrition, exercise, alcoholism, and seat belt use should be as of much concern and awareness as are diabetes, heart disease, and pneumonia. Primary-care physicians ought to be as comfortable counseling a bereaved widow as suturing the accident victim. They should be as comfortable teaching a young adult about birth control as they are revealing a diagnosis of dementia to an older adult. Primary-care physicians also should take greater responsibility for treating a larger percentage of their patients within the confines of their practice, and they should have greater skill in understanding which minority of patients need specialist care. This should, of course, all happen within a 15- to 20-minute visit and at a low cost to society. To do this, primary-care physicians must also be business managers, accountants, and entrepreneurs.

Amazingly, it is rare to find an example of the primary-care leadership making a concerted effort to say "enough is enough." On the contrary, primary care prides itself in this role as a giant receptacle—as being both the point of first contact and the final safety net.

We must wonder whether this acceptance of any responsibility deemed relevant to health is misguided. Suppose primary-care physicians were expected to teach adolescents advanced math skills, in addition to caring for their asthma and counseling them about smoking. Suppose primary-care physicians were expected to teach older adults how to advocate for public transportation systems, as well as counsel them that it was no longer safe to drive. Is the fact that most people come into contact with a primary-care doctor on a regular basis enough reason to heap this mountain of responsibilities on them? Is it possible to paralyze the system by assigning it a thousand roles? In the not-too-distant future, one might conceive of ameliorative (not curative) genetic engineering emerging as yet another role for primary care. Would we ask primary-care physicians to determine which children might be made more intelligent by a genetic manipulation? The issue here is that if primary care considers itself as open-ended, it will ineluctably move from curative (as it used to be) to preventive (as it is now) to ameliorative (as the future holds).

One response to the paralysis of the thousand roles has been to make the primary-care physician a quarterback, a gatekeeper, and a team leader—in other words, a care coordinator. In this role, the primary-care physician orchestrates patient care through a team of health-care providers that ranges from dieticians to specialty physicians to social workers. Unfortunately, this pushes many physicians away from the part of medicine they enjoy the most. It pushes the patient away from a part of medicine they seek: a patient–physician relationship. Another response has been to improve primary-care physicians' efficiency through electronic records, report cards, guidelines, continuous quality improvement, more examination rooms, performance indicators, and the full gamut of strategies for continuing medical education, ranging from lectures to recertification. Improved efficiency will never overcome the fundamental problem of having an inadequate capacity for meeting the level of expected productivity.

Although such strategies and many others result in incremental improvement in efficiency, all come at the cost of new issues, and none addresses the fundamental fact that primary care has limits. Primary-care in its current format cannot deliver what society seeks. Primary care physicians are unhappy about their ineffectiveness, their wheel-spinning, and their one-step-forward-two-steps-backward work style. This returns us to the "common dilemma" framed by Fry and Horder

(1994): The public and professional "wants" for health care will always be greater than the politically defined "needs" for health care, which, in turn, will always be greater than the national "resources" for health care.

With each new discovery, recommendation, expectation, and role, primary care becomes more ineffective. As primary care becomes more ineffective, more patients will seek care in alternative settings, and costs will increase. For those with the economic means, this might mean care from specialist physicians. For those without economic means, it may mean deferring care for prevention and chronic conditions, and perhaps even acute conditions. For a growing group of people, this might mean seeking care from alternative sources other than traditional allopathic medicine. In short, it is possible to render primary care practically ineffective. We can do this by feeding its appetite for new roles and new responsibilities. We argue that the "canary in the coalmine" for this paralysis of a thousand roles is the patient with emotional disorders.

One of the more impressive findings from this review of how depression has been reinvented over the past 50 years is the lack of substantial input, research, and leadership from primary-care physicians. Most of the current paradigm comes from specialty psychiatry or specialty psychiatrists working in primary care. In some respects, the pharmaceutical industry has played a greater role in developing the current treatment paradigm than have the physician–scientists who work in primary care. If emotional disorders were relatively rare, this passive role would be understandable and represent an appropriate allocation of a scarce resource. However, emotional disorders are among the most common reasons patients seek care in primary care. Why would the practitioners who know the most about the primary-care setting and the ways in which their patients seek care play such a small supporting role in developing care models? The answer may lie in the admonition given to psychiatry by Alan Gregg (1944), director for medical sciences at the Rockefeller Foundation, near the end of World War II:

My own formulation of your major limitations would be this: you are badly recruited, you are isolated from medicine, you are overburdened, and you are too inarticulate and long-suffering to secure redress from the public of some of the handicaps from which you and your patients suffer.

Primary-care physicians are overburdened, inarticulate, and long-suffering. They are poor lobbyists. The best evidence of the primary-care physicians' isolation from medicine is that they are receivers of knowledge and policy for their own practices and patients rather than producers.

The voice of primary-care physicians is heard only intermittently in the history of emotional disorders and typically only at times of extreme crisis identified by their patients. The minimal amount of research on emotional disorders that has been designed, directed, and interpreted by primary-care physicians is overshadowed by a much larger volume of research originating from other perspectives.

Only recently has the relevance of these other perspectives been questioned. In addition, the leadership of primary care has not consistently been involved in the highest levels of policy development. As such, the World Health Organization recommended the following:

General practitioners, clinical psychologists, and social workers, not at present sufficiently represented in the higher echelons of policy-making should be encouraged to seek representation for their disciplines on government bodies, so that their particular skills and perspectives can be used in the further planning of mental health services and primary care health care. (Working Group on First-Contact Mental Health Care 1984)

Continuing the Reinvention

If specialty psychiatry reaches out with a treatment model for depression in primary care that has important limitations, and if society places difficult expectations on primary care for treating depression, it is primary-care physicians' responsibility to respond with true leadership. Some public health advocates have suggested that primary care should assume a more community-based preventive health approach that focuses more effort not only on the medical determinants of disease but also on the genetic, social, and environmental determinants. Others have suggested that medicine's reach into private lives and social mores is already too intrusive. Primary care could do more to communicate its strengths and weaknesses and provide the leadership needed to emerge from the paralysis of a thousand roles.

To change this situation, the profession needs to invest substantial resources in building its capacity for participating in the solution. It must do this on a scale commensurate with the size and complexity of the problem of emotional disorders. There are three main components of this investment: *(1)* constructing primary-care laboratories that allow researchers access to the real world of primary care, *(2)* developing a stable cadre of primary-care researchers who practice in the setting where they conduct their research, and *(3)* developing a stable cadre of primary-care leaders and policy makers who can engage the public and the government leadership in securing resources for the first two components. These leaders also could facilitate societal discussion about primary care's scope and goals. The Royal College of General Practitioners, for example, has been active in this regard. Primary Care Trusts hold the money for a defined population and therefore can dictate to hospitals and specialists what they need and what they will purchase.

Investing in these three components—clinical laboratories, primary-care researchers, and primary-care leaders—is the only way to be certain that the next 50 years of reinventing depression will include the voices of primary-care physicians and patients. Simply developing this necessary infrastructure will take decades, and making changes in the primary-care system will take additional decades of work. This timeline is a reality even if a crisis, a fundamental discovery, or a massive redesign of the health-care system precipitates the change. We cannot continue to rely on these rare events. In the past 50 years, primary care has changed only in the face of one of these three major precipitants. If we put together the laboratory, the scientists, and the leaders, we can continually reinvent depression with less pain, cost, and misdirection than that witnessed over the past half-century. If we can accomplish this reinvention of depression, then this same laboratory, scientific team, and leadership will be healthy enough to reinvent primary care. This would be a great story to tell in 2050.

References

Akiskal HS, and WT McKinney Jr. 1975. Overview of recent research in depression: Integration of ten conceptual models into a comprehensive clinical frame. *Arch Gen Psychiatry* 32, no. 3: 285–305.

Allen FN, and M Kaufman. 1948. Nervous factors in general practice. *JAMA* 138: 1135–38.

Appel JW, and GW Beebe. 1946. Preventive psychiatry. *JAMA* 131: 1469–75.

Appel KE. 1954. Presidential address: The present challenge of psychiatry. *Am J Psychiatry* 111: 1–12.

Armstrong D. 1988. Historical origins of health behavior. In: R Anderson and JK Davies (eds.). *Health behavior research and health promotion.* Oxford: Oxford University Press.

———. 1994. *Outline of sociology as applied to medicine.* Oxford: Butterworth-Heinemann.

Aronowitz RA. 1998. *Making sense of illness: Science, society, and disease.* Cambridge: Cambridge University Press.

Attkisson CC, and JM Zich. 1990. *Depression in primary care: Screening and detection.* New York: Routledge.

Ayd FJ. 1961. *Recognizing the depression patient with essentials of management and treatment.* New York: Grune and Stratton.

Backett EM, JA Heady, and JCG Evans. 1954. Studies of a general practice: The doctor's job in an urban area. *Br Med J* i: 109–15.

Baehr G. 1950. Health insurance plan of Greater New York. *JAMA* 143: 637–40.

Balint M. 1957. *The doctor, his patient, and the illness.* London: Pitman Medical Publishing.

Ballenger JC, JR Davidson, Y Lecrubier, DJ Nutt, D Goldberg, KM Magruder, et al. 1999.

Consensus statement on the primary care management of depression from the International Consensus Group on Depression and Anxiety. *J Clin Psychiatry* 60, no. 7: S54–61.

Balter MB, J Levine, and DI Mannheimer. 1974. Cross-national study of the extent of anti-anxiety/sedative drug use. *N Engl J Med* 290: 769–74.

Banks MH, SAA Beresford, DC Morrell, JJ Waller, and CJ Watkins. 1975. Factors influencing demand for primary medical care in women aged 20–44 years. *Int J Epidemiol* 4: 189–95.

Barker DJP, and Osmond C. 1992. The maternal and infant origins of cardiovascular disease. In: M Marmot and P Elliot (eds.). *Coronary heart disease epidemiology*. Oxford: Oxford University Press.

Bartemeier LH, LS Kubie, KA Menniger, J Romano, and Whitehorn JC. 1946. Combat exhaustion. *J Nerv Ment Dis* 104: 358–89, 489–525.

Bauer J. 1953. Principles of psychotherapy in general practice. *Ann Intern Med* 39: 81–91.

Bebbington R. 1969. A review of 508 consecutive patients seen in general practice. *J R Coll Gen Pract* 18: 27.

Beck AT. 1962. Reliability of psychiatric diagnoses: A critique of systematic studies. *Am J Psychiatry* 119: 210–16.

Bedford S. 1987. *Aldous Huxley: A biography*. London: Paladin Grafton Books.

Berrios GE. 1983. Anxiolytic drugs. In: GE Berrios and JH Dowson (eds.). *Treatment and management in adult psychiatry* (pp. 3–29). London: Bailliere Tindall.

———. 1985. The psychopathology of affectivity: Conceptual and historical aspects. *Psychol Med* 15: 745–58.

———. 1988. Historical background to abnormal psychology. In: E Miller and P Cooper (eds.). *Adult abnormal psychology* (pp. 26–51). London: Churchill Livingstone.

———. 1992. The history of affective disorders. In: ES Paykel (ed.). *Handbook of affective disorders,* 2nd ed. (pp. 43–56). London: Churchill Livingstone.

———. 1994. Historiography of mental symptoms and disease. *Hist Psychiatry* 5: 175–90.

———. 1996. *History of mental symptoms: The history of descriptive psychopathology since the 19th century.* Cambridge: Cambridge University Press.

———. 1997. The scientific origins of electroconvulsive therapy. *Hist Psychiatry* 8: 105–19.

———. 1999a. Anxiety disorders: A conceptual history. *J Affect Disord* 56: 83–94.

———. 1999b. Classification in psychiatry: A conceptual history. *Aust N Z J Psychiatry* 33: 145–60.

———. 2000. The history of psychiatric concepts. In FA Henn et al. (eds.). *Foundations of psychiatry* (pp. 1–30). Heidelberg: Springer.

Berrios GE, and A Bulbena-Villarasa. 1990. The Hamilton Depression Scale and the numerical description of the symptoms of depression. In: P Bech and A. Coppen (eds.). *The Hamilton scales.* Berlin: Springer-Verlag.

Berrios GE, and E Chen. 1993. Symptom-recognition and neural-networks. *Br J Psychiatry* 163: 308–14.

Berrios GE, and IS Markova. 2002a. Assessment and measurement in neuropsychiatry: A conceptual history. *Semin Clin Neuropsychiatry* 7: 3–10.

———. 2002b. Biological psychiatry: Conceptual issues. In: H D'Haenen, JA den Boer, and P Willner (eds.). *Biological psychiatry* (pp. 3–24). New York: John Wiley.

Berrios GE and R Porter (eds.). 1995. *A history of clinical psychiatry.* London: Athlone Press.

Bertalanffy LV. 1968. *General systems theory: Foundations, development, applications.* New York: George Braziller.

Berwick DM. 1998. Developing and testing changes in delivery of care. *Ann Intern Med* 128: 651–56.

Bevan A. 1948. A message to the medical profession from the Minister of Health. *Br Med J* ii: 1.

Bierring WL. 1934. The family doctor and the changing order: President's address. *JAMA* 102: 1995–98.

Billings AG, and Moos RH. 1982. Psychosocial theory and research on depression: An integrative framework and review. *Clin Psychol Rev* 2: 213–37.

Blacker C, and A. Clare. 1987. Depressive disorder in primary care. *Br J Psychiatry* 150: 737–51.

Blackwell B. 1973. Psychotropic drugs in use today: The role of diazepam in medical practice. *JAMA* 225: 1637–41.

Blendon R, R Letiman, I Morrison, and K Donelan. 1990. Satisfaction with health systems in ten nations. *Health Aff* 9: 185–92.

Blendon RJ, K Donelan, R Leitman, et al. 1993. Physicians' perspectives on caring for patients in the United States, Canada, and West Germany. *N Engl J Med* 14: 1011–16.

Blendon, RJ, J Benson, K Donelan, R Leitman, H Taylor, C Koeck, and D Gitterman. 1995. Who has the best health care system? A second look. *Health Aff* 14: 220–30.

Bloor D. 1991. *Knowledge and social imagery.* Chicago: University of Chicago Press.

Bosanquet N, and C Salisbury. 1998. The practice. In: I Loudon, J Horder, and C Webster (eds.). *General practice under the national health service 1948–1997.* London: Clarendon Press.

Bradshaw D. 1994. Introduction to *Brave New World* by A Huxley. London: Flamingo.

Broadhead WE, DG Blazer, LK George, and CK Tse. 1990. Depression, disability days and days lost from work in a prospective epidemiologic survey. *JAMA* 264, no. 19: 2524–28.

Brodman K, AJ Erdman, I Lorge, CP Gershenson, and HG Wolff. 1952. The Cornell Medical Index–Health Questionnaire: The evaluation of emotional disturbances. *J Clin Psychol* 8: 119–24.

Brody DS, CE Lerman, HG Wolfson, and GC Caputo. 1990. Improvement in physicians' counseling of patients with mental health problems. *Arch Intern Med* 150: 993–98.

Brotherstone JHF, and SPW Chave. 1956. General practice on a new housing estate. *Br J Prev Soc Med* 10: 200–207.

Brown JH. 1979. Suicide in Britain: More attempts, fewer deaths, lessons for public policy. *Arch Gen Psychiatry* 36: 1119–24.

Brown M. 1947. The recognition and management of depressed mental states. *Ill Med J* August: 95–99.

Bury M. 1996. Caveat venditor: Social dimensions of a medical controversy. In: D Healy and P Declan (eds.). *Psychotropic drug development.* London: Chapman and Hall.

Cade JFJ. 1949. Lithium salts in the treatment of psychotic excitement. *Med J Aust* 36: 349–52.

Callahan CM. 2001. Quality improvement research on late life depression in primary care. *Med Care* 39: 772–84.

Callahan CM, HC Hendrie, and WM Tierney. 1996. The recognition and treatment of late life depression: A view from primary care. *Int J Psychiatry Med* 26: 155–71.

Cartwright A. 1967. *Patients and their doctors. A study of general practice.* London: Routledge and Kegan Paul.

Cartwright A, and R Anderson. 1981. *General practice revisited: A second study of patients and their doctors.* London: Tavistock Publications.

Cartwright A, and R Marshall. 1965. General practice in 1963. *Med Care* 3: 69–87.

Chain EB. 1963. Academic and industrial contributions to drug research. *Nature* 200: 441–53.

Cole JO. 1964. Therapeutic efficacy of antidepressant drugs: A review. *JAMA* 190: 448–55.

Cole MG, F Bellavance, and A Mansour. 1999. Prognosis of depression in elderly community and primary care populations: A systematic review and meta-analysis. *Am J Psychiatry* 156, no. 8: 1182–89.

Collings JS. 1950. General practice in England today. *Lancet* i: 555–85.

Collins SD. 1940. Cases and days of illness among males and females with special reference to confinement to bed. *Public Health Rep* (U.S. Public Health Service) 55: 47–93.

Conwell Y, K Olsen, ED Caine, and C Flannery. 1991. Suicide in late life: Psychological autopsy findings. *Int Psychogeriatr* 3: 59–66.

Cooper JE. 1986. Discussant. In: M Shepherd, G Wilkinson, and P Williams (eds.). *Mental illness in primary care settings.* London: Tavistock Publications.

Cooper JE, RE Kendell, BJ Gurland, L Sharpe, JRM Copeland, and R Simon. 1972. *Psychiatric diagnosis in New York and London.* London: Oxford University Press.

Coulehan JL, HC Schulberg, MR Block, MJ Madonia, and E Rodriguez. 1997. Treating depressed primary care patients improves their physical, mental, and social functioning. *Arch Intern Med* 157: 1113–20.

Dawber TR. 1980. *The Framingham study: The epidemiology of atherosclerotic disease.* Cambridge: Harvard University Press.

deGruy FV, and H Pincus. 1996. The DSM-IV-PC: A manual for diagnosing mental disorders in the primary care setting. *J Am Board Fam Pract* 9: 274–81.

Densen PM, E Balamuth, and NR Deardorff. 1960. Medical care plans as a source of morbidity data: Prevalence of illness and associated volume of services. *Milbank Q* 38: 48–101.

DeNuzzo RV. 1979. Annual Albany College of Pharmacy prescription survey. *Medical Marketing and Media* 14: 17–37.

Department of Health and Human Services. 1999. *Mental health: A report of the surgeon general—executive summary.* Rockville, MD: U.S. Department of Health and Human Services, Substance Abuse and Mental Health Services Administration, Center for Mental Health Services, National Institutes of Health, National Institute of Mental Health.

Depression Guideline Panel. 1993. *Depression in primary care:* Vol. 2. *Treatment of major depression.* Clinical Practice Guidelines No. 5. AHCPR Publication No. 93-0551. Rockville, MD: U.S. Department of Health and Human Services, Public Health Service.

Dew MA, EJ Bromet, D Brent, and JB Greenhouse. 1987. A quantitative literature review of the effectiveness of suicide prevention centers. *J Consult Clin Psychol* 55: 239–44.

Diagnostic and statistical manual of mental disorders: DSM-IV. 4th ed. 1994. Washington, DC: American Psychiatric Association.

Diekstra RFW. 1995. The epidemiology of suicide and parasuicide. In: RFW Diekstra, W Gulbinat, I Kienhorst, and D de Leo (eds.). *Preventive strategies on suicide.* Leiden: E. J. Brill.

Diekstra RFW, and M van Egmond. 1989. Suicide and attempted suicide in general practice, 1979–1985. *Acta Psychiatr Scand* 79: 268–75.

Donelan K, RJ Blendon, C Schoen, K Davis, and K Binns. 1999. The cost of health system change: Public discontent in five nations. *Health Aff* 18: 206–16.

Downes J. 1950. Causes of illness among males and females. *Milbank Q* 28: 407–28.

Downes J, and K Simon. 1954. Characteristics of psychoneurotic patients and their families as revealed in a general morbidity study. *Milbank Q* 32: 42–60.

Duffy J. 1993. *From humors to medical science: A history of American medicine*, 2nd ed. Urbana: University of Illinois Press.

Duggan CF. 1997. Course and outcome of depression. In: A Honig and HM van Praag (eds.). *Depression: Neurobiological, psychopathological and therapeutic advances.* Chichester: John Wiley and Sons.

Dunlop D. 1970. The use and abuse of psychotropic drugs. *Proc R Soc Med* 63: 1279–82.

Dunlop DM, TL Henderson, and RS Inch. 1952. A survey of 17,301 prescriptions on Form E.C.10. *Br Med J* i: 292–95.

Editorial [unsigned]. 1970. Psychiatric disorders in the community. *Br Med J* 2: 435.

Eimerl TS, and RJ Pearson. 1966. Working-time in general practice: How general practitioners use their time. *Br Med J* 2, no. 529: 1549–54.

Eisenberg L. 1992. Treating depression and anxiety in primary care: Closing the gap between knowledge and practice. *N Engl J Med* 16: 1080–84.

Elkin I, MT Shea, JT Watkins, SD Imber, SM Sotsky, JF Collin, DR Glass, PA Pilkonis, WR Leber, JP Docherty, et al. 1989. National Institute of Mental Health Treatment of Depression Collaborative Research Program: General effectiveness of treatments. *Arch Gen Psychiatry* 46: 971–82.

Elkin I, RD Gibbons, MT Shea, SM Sotsky, JT Watkins, PA Pilkonis, and D Hedeker. 1995. Initial severity and differential treatment outcome in the National Institute of Mental Health Treatment of Depression Collaborative Research Program. *J Consult Clin Psychol* 63: 841–47.

Farber IE. 1975. Sane and insane: Constructions and misconstructions. *J Abnorm Psychol* 84: 589–620.

Featherstone RM, and A Simon. 1959. *A pharmacologic approach to the study of the mind.* Springfield, IL: Charles C. Thomas.

Feighner JP, E Robins, SB Guze, RA Woodruff, G Winokur, and R Munoz. 1972. Diagnostic criteria for use in psychiatric research. *Arch Gen Psychiatry* 26: 57–63.

Ferrier SE. 1824. *The inheritance.* Edinburgh: Blackwood.

Ferris P. 1967. *The doctors.* London: Harmondsworth Penguin Books.

Fink R, SS Goldensohn, S Shapiro, and EF Daily. 1967. Treatment of patients designated by family doctors as having emotional problems. *Am J Public Health* 57: 1550–64.

Fournier R, and Neergaard L. Records show McCaim in 'good' health. *Associated Press.* Dec 6, 1999.

Friedland J, and M McColl. 1992. Disability and depression: Some etiological considerations. *Soc Sci Med* 4: 395–403.

Frierson RL. 1991. Suicide attempts by the old and the very old. *Arch Intern Med* 151: 141–44.

Fry J. 1952. A year of general practice: A study in morbidity. *Br Med J* ii: 249–52.

———. 1957. Five years of general practice; a study in simple epidemiology. *Br Med J* 29: 1453–7.

———. 1966. *Profiles of disease: A study in the natural history of common diseases.* Edinburgh: E & S Livingtone.

———. 1974. *Common diseases: Their nature, incidence and care.* Lancaster: Medical and Technical Publishing.

————. 1979. *Common diseases: Their nature, incidence and care*, 2nd ed. Lancaster: MTP Press.

————. 1982. Psychiatric illness in general practice. In: AW Clare and M Lader (eds.). *Psychiatry and general practice*. London: Academic Press.

————. 1988. *General practice and primary health care, 1940s–1980s*. London: Nuffield Provincial Hospital Trust.

Fry J, and J Horder. 1994. *Primary health care in an international context*. London: Nuffield Provincial Hospital Trust.

Fry J, D Light, J Rodnick, and P Orton. 1995. *Reviving primary care: A US–UK comparison*. Oxford: Radcliffe Medical Press.

Gabe J. 1991. *Understanding tranquilizer use*. London: Tavistock/Routledge.

Gabe J, and P Williams. 1986. *Tranquilizers: Social, psychological, and clinical perspectives*. London: Tavistock.

General Medical Services Committee. 1965. Report of the General Medical Services Committee. *Br Med J* ii(suppl.): 176–90.

Gibson R. 1981. *The family doctor: His life and history*. London: George Allen and Unwin.

Gifford EG. 1973. Fildes and "The Doctor." *JAMA* 224: 61–63.

Goethe JW, BL Szarek, and WL Cook. 1988. A comparison of adequately vs. inadequately treated depressed inpatients. *J Nerv Ment Dis* 176: 465–70.

Goldberg D, and B Blackwell. 1970. Psychiatric illness in general practice. *British Med J* 2: 439–43.

Goldberg D, and P Huxley. 1980. *Mental illness in the community: The pathway to psychiatric care*. London: Tavistock.

————. 1992. *Common mental disorders: A bio-social model*. London: Tavistock/Routledge.

Goldberg D, M Privett, B Ustun, G Simon, and M Linden. 1998. The effects of detection and treatment on the outcome of major depression in primary care: A naturalistic study in 15 cities. *Br J Gen Pract* 48: 1840–44.

Gorman Mike. 1956. *Every other bed*. Cleveland: World Publishing.

Greenberg RP, RF Bornstein, MD Greenberg, and S Fisher. 1992. A meta-analysis of antidepressant outcome under "blinder" conditions. *J Consult Clin Psychol* 60: 664–69.

Gregg A. 1944. A critique of psychiatry. *Am J Psychiatry* 101: 285–91.

Grinker RR. 1977. The inadequacies of contemporary psychiatric diagnosis. In: VM Rakoff, HC Stancer, and HB Kedward (eds.). *Psychiatric diagnosis*. New York: Brunner/Mazel.

Grob GN. 1994. *The mad among us*. New York: Free Press.

Gulbinat W. 1995. The epidemiology of suicide in old age. In: RFW Diekstra, W Gulbinat, I Kienhorst, and D de Leo (eds.). *Preventive strategies on suicide*. Leiden: E. J. Brill.

Gurin G, J Veroff, and S Feld. 1960. *Americans view their mental health: A nationwide interview survey*. New York: Basic Books.

Gurland BJ, J Copeland, J Kuriansky, M Kelleher, L Sharpe, and LL Dean. 1983. *The mind and mood of aging: Mental health problems of the community elderly in New York and London*. New York: Croom Helm; London: Haworth Press.

Haggerty RJ. 1963. Etiology of decline in general practice. *JAMA* 185: 179–82.

Hart JT. 1994. *Feasible socialism: The National Health Service, past, present, and future*. London: Socialist Health Association.

Healy D. 1997. *The antidepressant era*. Cambridge: Harvard University Press.

Heller J. 1962. *Catch-22*. London: Jonathan Cape.

Himmelwert F. 1960. *The collected papers of Paul Ehrlich*. London: Pergamon.

Himwich H. 1958. Psychopharmacologic drugs. *Science* 127: 59–71.

Hoeper EW, GR Nycz, LG Kessler, JD Burke Jr, and WE Pierce. 1984. The usefulness of screening for mental illness. *Lancet* 33–35.

Hoff P. 1995. Kraepelin. In: GE Berrios and R Porter (eds.). *A history of clinical psychiatry*. London: Athlone Press.

Hoffman C, D Rice, and HY Sung. 1996. Persons with chronic conditions: Their prevalence and costs. *JAMA* 276: 1473–79.

Hoffman NY. 1972. The doctor as scapegoat: A study in ambivalence. *JAMA* 220: 58–61.

Hollingsworth JR. 1986. *A political economy of medicine: Great Britain and the United States*. Baltimore: Johns Hopkins University Press.

Hollister LE. 1972. Mental disorders: antianxiety and antidepressant drugs. *N Engl J Med* 286: 1195–98.

Honig A, and HM van Praag. 1997. *Depression: Neurobiological, psychopathological and therapeutic advances*. Chichester: John Wiley and Sons.

Honigsbaum F. 1979. *The division in British medicine: A history of the separation of general practice from hospital care: 1911–1948*. London: Kogan Page.

Horder J. 1954. Illness in general practice. *Practitioner* 173: 172–87.

———. 1991. Long-term tranquilizer use: A general practitioner's view. In: J Gabe (ed.). *Understanding tranquilizer use*. London: Tavistock/Routledge.

———. 1998. Developments in other countries. In: I Loudon, J Horder, and C. Webster (eds.). *General practice under the National Health Service, 1948–1997*. London: Clarendon Press.

Howard CRG. 1959. The problem of defining the extent of morbidity in general practice. *J R Coll Gen Pract* 2: 119.

Hull FM. 1981. International sore throats. *J R Coll Gen Pract* 31: 45–48.

Huntley RR. 1963. Epidemiology of family practice. *JAMA* 185: 175–78.

Huxley A. 1959a. *Brave New World Revisited*. London: Chatto and Windus.

———. 1959b. The final revolution. In: RM Featherstone and A Simon (eds). *A pharmacologic approach to the study of the mind*. Springfield, IL: Charles C. Thomas.

———. 1994. *Brave New World*. London: Flamingo. Originally published in 1932 by Chatto and Windus, London.

Imber SD, PA Pilkonis, SM Sotsky, I Elkin, JT Watkins, JF Collins, MT Shea, WR Leber, and DR Glass. 1990. Mode-specific effects among three treatments for depression. *J Consult Clin Psychol* 58: 352–59.

International Statistical Classification of Diseases and Related Health Problems, 1989 Revision, Geneva, World Health Organization, 1992.

Jeffreys M. 1973. Medicine takers. *J R Coll Gen Pract* 23(suppl 2): 9–11.

Jeffreys M, JHF Brothestone, and A Cartwright. 1960. Consumption of medicines on a working class housing estate. *Br J Prev Soc Med* 14: 64–76.

Johnson DAW. 1974. A study of antidepressant medication in general practice. *Br J Psychiatry* 125: 186–92.

Johnson FN. 1984. *The history of lithium therapy*. London: Macmillan.

Johnson WM. 1946. Will the family doctor survive? *JAMA* 132: 1–4.

Johnstone A, and D Goldberg. 1976. Psychiatric screening in general practice: A controlled trial. *Lancet* 20: 605–8.

Johnstone EC, DG Cunningham-Owens, CD Frith, K McPherson, C Dowie, G Riley, and A Gold. 1980. Neurotic illness and its response to anxiolytic and antidepressant treatment. *Psychol Med* 10: 321–29.

Kannel WB. 1992. The Framingham experience. In: M Marmot, and P Elliot (eds.). *Coronary heart disease epidemiology*. Oxford: Oxford University Press.

Kannel WB, and M Larson. 1993. Long-term epidemiologic prediction of coronary artery disease: The Framingham experience. *Cardiology* 82: 137–52.

Katon WJ. Psychiatry and primary care. 1991. *Gen Hosp Psychiatry* 13: 9.

Katon W, and H Schulberg. 1992. Epidemiology of depression in primary care. *Gen Hosp Psychiatry* 14: 237–47.

Katon W, M Von Korff, EHB Lin, E Walker, GE Simon, T Bush, P Robinson, and J Russo. 1995. Collaborative management to achieve treatment guidelines. *JAMA* 273: 1026–31.

Katz IR, and GS Alexopoulos. 1996. Consensus Update Conference: Diagnosis and treatment of late life depression. Proceedings of the Geriatric Psychiatry Alliance. *Am J Geriatr Psychiatry* 4, no. 4: S1–S2.

Katzelnick DJ, GE Simon, SD Pearson, WG Manning, CP Helstad, HJ Henk, SM Cole, EH Lin, LH Taylor, and KA Kobak. 2000. Randomized trial of a depression management program in high utilizers of medical care. *Arch Fam Med* 9: 345–51.

Kaufman MR, and S Bernstein. 1957. A psychiatric evaluation of the problem patient. *JAMA* 163: 108–11.

Kaufman SR. 1993. *The healer's tale: Transforming medicine and culture*. Madison, Wis: University of Wisconsin Press.

Kedward HB, and B Cooper. 1966. Neurotic disorders in urban practice: A three-year follow-up. *J Coll Gen Pract* 12: 148–63.

Keller MB, and PW Lavori. 1988. The adequacy of treating depression. *J Nerv Ment Dis* 176: 471–74.

Keller MB, GL Klerman, PW Lavori, JA Fawcett, W Coryell, and J Endicott. 1982. Treatment received by depressed patients. *JAMA* 248: 1848–55.

Keller MB, GL Lerman, PW Lavori, W Coryell, J Endicott, and J Taylor. 1984. Long-term outcomes of episodes of major depression: Clinical and public health significance. *JAMA* 252: 788–92.

Keller MB, PW Lavori, GL Klerman, NC Andreasen, J Endicott, W Coryell, J Fawcett, JP Rice, and RM Hirschfeld. 1986. Low levels and lack of predictors of somatotherapy and psychotherapy received by depressed patients. *Arch Gen Psychiatry* 43: 458–66.

Kendell RE. 1975. *The role of diagnosis in psychiatry*. Oxford: Blackwell.

Kendell RE, JE Cooper, AJ Gourlay, JRM Copeland, L Sharpe, and BJ Gurland. 1971. Diagnostic criteria of American and British psychiatrists. *Arch Gen Psychiatry* 25: 123–30.

Kennedy GJ. 1996. *Suicide and depression in late life*. New York: John Wiley and Sons.

Kessel N, and M Shepherd. 1962. Neurosis in hospital and general practice. *J Ment Sci* 108: 159.

Kickbusch I. 1988. Introduction. In: R Anderson and JK Davies (eds.). *Health Behavior Research and Health Promotion*. Oxford: Oxford University Press.

Kleinman A, L Eisenberg, and B Good. 1978. Culture, illness, and care. *Ann Intern Med* 88: 251–58.

Kline NS. 1964. The practical management of depression. *JAMA* 190: 732–40.

Kornitzer M. 1992. Changing individual behaviour. In: M Marmot and P Elliot (eds.). *Coronary heart disease epidemiology*. Oxford: Oxford University Press.

Kramarow E, H Lentzner, R Rooks, J Weeks, and S Saydah. 1999. *Health and aging chartbook: Health, United States, 1999*. Hyattsville, MD: National Center for Health Statistics.

Kramer PD. 1993. *Listening to Prozac.* New York: Penguin Books.

Kuhn R. 1958. The treatment of depressive states with G 22355 (imipramine hydrochloride). *Am J Psychiatry* 115: 459–64.

Lader M. 1996. The rise and fall of the benzodiazepines. In: D Healy and P Doogan (eds.). *Psychotropic drug development.* London: Chapman and Hall.

Lain Entralgo P. 1969. *Doctor and patient.* London: Weidenfeld and Nicholson.

Lebowitz BD, JL Pearson, LS Schneider, et al. 1997. Diagnosis and treatment of depression in late life: Consensus statement update. *JAMA* 278: 1186–90.

Lees DS, and MH Cooper. 1963. The work of the general practitioner: An analytical survey of studies of general practice. *J R Coll Gen Pract* 6: 408.

Le Fanu J. 1999. *The rise and fall of modern medicine.* London: Little, Brown.

Lehmann HE. 1960. Combined pharmaco-fever treatment with imipramine and typhoid vaccine in the management of depressive conditions. *Am J Psychiatry* 117: 356–58.

Lemere F. 1957. Treatment of mild depression in general office practice. *JAMA* 164: 516–18.

Lennard HL, LJ Epstein, A Bernstein, and DC Ransom. 1970. Hazards implicit in prescribing psychoactive drugs. *Science* 169: 438–41.

Lester D. 1995. Preventing suicide by restricting access to methods for suicide. In: RFW Diekstra, W Gulbinat, I Kienhorst, and D de Leo (eds.). *Preventive strategies on suicide.* Leiden: E. J. Brill.

Lew EA. 1973. High blood pressure, other risk factors, and longevity. *Am J Med* 55: 281–94.

Lewis A. 1942. Incidence of neurosis in England under war conditions. *Lancet* i: 175–83.

———. 1945. On the place of physical treatment in psychiatry. *Br Med Bull* 3: 614.

———. 1953. Health as a social concept. *Br J Sociol* 4: 109–24.

Lin EH, WJ Katon, GE Simon, M Von Korff, TM Bush, CM Rutter, et al. 1997. Achieving guidelines for the treatment of depression in primary care: Is physician education enough? *Med Care* 35: 831–42.

Lin EH, GE Simon, WJ Katon, JE Russo, M Von Korff, TM Bush, et al. 1999. Can enhanced acute-phase treatment of depression improve long-term outcomes? A report of randomized trials in primary care. *Am J Psychiatry* 156: 643–45.

Linn LS, and J Yager. 1980. The effect of screening, sensitization, and feedback on notation of depression. *J Med Educ* 55: 942–49.

Logan WPD, and EM Brooke. 1957. *Studies on medical and population subjects:* No. 12. *The survey of sickness 1943–52.* London: HMSO.

Macfarlane G. 1979. *Howard Florey: The making of a great scientist.* Oxford: Oxford University Press.

———. 1984. *Alexander Fleming: The man and the myth.* London: Chatto and Windus.

Magruder-Habib K, WWK Zung, and JR Feussner, 1990. Improving physicians' recognition and treatment of depression in general medical care. *Med Care* 28: 239–50.

Malamud M. 1959. *The range of therapeutic results from various methods of treatment.* A pharmacologic approach to the study of the mind. In: RM Featherstone and A Simon (ed.). Springfield, IL: Charles C. Thomas.

Marinker M. 1998. "What is wrong" and "How we know it": Changing concepts of illness in general practice. In: I Loudon, J Horder, and C Webster (eds.). *General practice under the National Health Service, 1948–1997.* Oxford: Clarendon Press.

Marr HC. 1919. *Psychoses of the war.* London: Oxford Medical Publications.

Marsh GN, RB Wallace, and J Whewell. 1976. Anglo-American contrasts in general practice. *Br. Med J* i: 1321–25.

McDonald CJ, WM Tierney, DK Martin, and JM Overhage. 1992. The Regenstrief Medical Record System: 20 years experience in hospital outpatient clinics and neighborhood health centers. *MD Computing* 9: 206–17.

McDonald CJ, JM Overhage, WM Tierney, et al. 1999. The Regenstrief Medical Record System: A quarter century experience. *Int J Med Inf* 54: 225–53.

McGinnis JM, and WH Foege. 1993. Actual causes of death in the United States. *JAMA* 270: 2207–12.

McKeown T. 1961. The next forty years in public health. *Milbank Q* 39: 594–630.

McWhinney IR. 1966. General practice as an academic discipline. *Lancet* i: 419–23.

Mechanic D. 1972. General medical practice: Some comparisons between the work of primary care physicians in the United States and England and Wales. *Med Care* 10: 402–20.

Menninger K. 1963. *The vital balance: The life process in mental health and illness.* New York: Viking Press.

Menninger WC. 1947a. The problem of the neurotic patient. *Ann Intern Med* 27: 487–93.

———. 1947b. Psychiatric experience in the war. *Am J Psychiatry* 103: 577–86.

———. 1948. *Psychiatry: Its evolution and present status.* Ithaca, NY: Cornell University Press.

Mintz M. 1965. *The therapeutic nightmare.* Boston: Houghton Mifflin.

Montagne M. 1991. The culture of long-term tranquilizer users. In: J Gabe (ed.). *Understanding tranquilizer use.* London: Tavistock/Routledge.

Moore HH. 1927. *American medicine and the people's health.* New York: D. Appleton.

Morrell D. 1998. Introduction and overview. In: I Loudon, J Horder, and C Webster (eds.). *General practice under the National Health Service, 1948–1997.* London: Clarendon Press.

Murphy GE, and RD Wetzel. 1980. Suicide risk by birth cohort in the United States, 1949 to 1974. *Arch Gen Psychiatry* 37: 519–23.

Murray CJ, and AD Lopez. 1996. *The global burden of disease: A comprehensive assessment of mortality and disability from diseases, injuries and risk factors in 1990 and projected to 2020.* Cambridge, MA: Harvard School of Public Health on behalf of the World Health Organization and the World Bank.

Mynors-Wallis LM, DH Gath, AR Lloyd-Thomas, and D Tomlinson. 1995. Randomised controlled trial comparing problem solving treatment with amitriptyline and placebo for major depression in primary care. *Br Med J* 310: 441–45.

Nemeroff CB. 1998. The neurobiology of depression. *Sci Am* Jun; 278(6): 42–9.

Nestler EJ, E Gould, H Husseini, et al. 2002. Preclinical models: Status of basic research in depression. *Biol Psychiatry* 52: 503–28.

New York Times. 1905. Celebrate Mark Twain's Seventieth Birthday. December 6.

Nuki G. 1999. Osteoarthritis: A problem of joint failure. *Z Rheumatol* 58: 142–47.

Numbers RL. 1979. The third party. In: MJ Vogel and CE Rosenberg (eds.). *The therapeutic revolution.* Philadephia: University of Pennsylvania Press.

Oldham PD, G Pickering, JA Roberts, and GS Sowry. 1960. The nature of essential hypertension. *Lancet* 1: 1085–93.

Ormel J, A Brilman E, and W van den Brink. 1993. Outcome of depression and anxiety in primary care: A three-wave 3.5 year study of psychopathology and disability. *Arch Gen Psychiatry* 50: 759–66.

Parish PA. 1971. The prescribing of psychotropic drugs in general practice. *J R Coll Gen Pract* 21(suppl 4): 1–77.

————. 1973. Medical use of psychotropic drugs. *J R Coll Gen Pract* 23(suppl 2): 49–58.

————. 1982. The use of psychotropic drugs in general practice. In: AW Clare and M Lader (eds.). *Psychiatry and general practice.* London: Academic Press.

Parry HJ, MB Balter, GD Mellinger, IH Cisin, and DI Manheimer. 1973. National patterns of psychotherapeutic drug use. *Arch Gen Psychiatry* 28: 769–83.

Pasamanick B, DW Roberts, PV Lemkau, and DE Krugeger. 1957. A survey of mental disease in an urban population: Prevalence by age, sex, and severity of impairment. *Am J Public Health* 47, no. 8: 923–29.

Pasamanick B, S Dinitz, and M Lefton. 1959. Psychiatric orientation and its relation to diagnosis and treatment in a mental hospital. *Am J Psychiatry* 116: 127–32.

Paykel ES, and RG Priest. 1992. Recognition and management of depression in general practice: Consensus statement. *Br Med J* 305: 1198–202.

Paykel ES, A Tylee, A Wright, RG Priest, S Rix, and D Hart. 1997. The Defeat Depression Campaign: Psychiatry in the public arena. *Am J Psychiatry* 154(suppl 6): 59–65.

Pellegrino ED. 1979. The sociocultural impact of 20th century therapeutics. In: MJ Vogel and E Rosenberg (eds.). *The therapeutic revolution.* Philadelphia: University of Pennsylvania Press.

Pemberton J. 1949. Illness in general practice. *Br Med J* i: 306–8.

Peterson OL, LP Andrews, RS Spain, and BG Greenberg. 1956. An analytical study of North Carolina general practice, 1953–1954. *J Med Educ* December: 1–165.

Pinchot PJ. 1997. DSM-III and its reception: A European view. *Am J Psychiatry* 154(suppl 6): 47–54.

Postel-Vinay N. 1996. *A century of arterial hypertension.* Chichester: John Wiley and Sons.

Prather JE. 1991. Decoding advertising: The role of communication studies in explaining the popularity of minor tranquilizers. In: J Gabe (ed.). *Understanding tranquilizer use.* London: Tavistock/Routledge.

Quill TE, CK Cassel, and DE Meier. 1992. Care of the hopelessly ill: Proposed criteria for physician assisted suicide. *N Engl J Med* 327: 1380–84.

Rakoff VM, HC Stancer, and HB Kedward. 1977. *Psychiatric diagnosis.* New York: Brunner/Mazel.

Rand EH, LW Badger, and DR Coggins. 1988. Toward a resolution of contradictions: Utility of feedback from the GHQ. *Gen Hosp Psych* 10: 189–96.

Randolph E. 1988. At first rumor percolated, then it surfaced. *Washington Post.* 4 August.

Rees JR. 1945. *The shaping of psychiatry by war.* New York: W.W. Norton.

Regier DA, ID Goldberg, and CA Taube. 1978. The de facto U.S. mental health services system. *Arch Gen Psychiatry* 35: 658–93.

Regier DA, RMA Hirshfield, FK Goodwin, JD Burke, JB Lozar, and LL Judd. 1988. The NIMH Depression Awareness, Recognition, and Treatment Program: Structure, aims, and scientific basis. *Am J Psychiatry* 145: 1351–57.

Rennie TAC. 1946. What can the practitioner do in treating neuroses? *Bull New York Acad Med* 22: 23–37.

Report of the General Practice Review Committee. 1953. A review of general practice, 1951–1952. *Br Med J* Suppl: 131–54.

Research Unit in Health and Behavioral Change, University of Edinburgh. 1989. *Changing the public health.* Chichester: John Wiley and Sons.

Revicki DA, GE Simon, K Chan, W Katon, and J Heiligenstein. 1998. Depression, health-related quality of life, and medical cost outcomes of receiving recommended levels of antidepressant treatment. *J Fam Pract* 47: 446–52.

Richards AN. 1964. Production of penicillin in the United States, 1941–46. *Nature* 201: 441–45.

Ridenour N. 1961. *Mental health in the United States: A fifty-year history.* Cambridge, MA: Harvard University Press.

Risch SC. 1997. Recent advances in depression research: From stress to molecular biology and brain imaging. *J Clin Psychiatry* 58(Suppl 5): 3–6.

Robins LN, and DA Regier. 1991. *Psychiatric disorders in America.* New York: Free Press.

Robins LN, JK Wing, HU Wittchen, JE Helzer, TF Babor, J Burke, A Farmer, A Jablensky, R Pickens, DA Regier, N Sartorius, and LH Towle. 1994. The Composite International Diagnostic Interview. In: JE Mezzich, MR Jorge, and IM Salloum (eds.). *Psychiatric epidemiology.* Baltimore: Johns Hopkins University Press.

Robinson D. 1978. *The miracle finders: The stories behind the most important breakthroughs of modern medicine.* London: Robson Books.

Rodney RM. 1993. *Mark Twain overseas.* Washington DC: Three Continents Press.

Rose G. 1985. Sick individuals and sick populations. *Int J Epidemiol* 14: 32–38.

———. 1992. Strategies of prevention: The individual and the population. In: M Marmot and P Elliot (eds.). *Coronary heart disease epidemiology.* Oxford: Oxford University Press.

Rosenhan DL. 1973. On being sane in insane places. *Science* 179: 250–58.

Roth M. 1990. Max Hamilton: A life devoted to psychiatric science. In: P Bech and A Coppen (eds.). *The Hamilton scales.* Berlin: Springer-Verlag.

Roth M, and C Mountjoy. 1990. Lines of demarcation and continuity between the anxiety and depressive disorders. In: B Leonard and P Spencer (eds.). *Antidepressants: Thirty years on.* London: Clinical Neuroscience Publishers.

Rothman DJ. 1997. *Beginnings count: The technological imperative in American health care.* New York: Oxford University Press.

Rudolf GDM. 1949. The treatment of depression with desoxyephedrine. *J Ment Sci* 95: 920–929.

Sainsbury P. 1986. Depression, suicide, and suicide prevention. In: A Roy (ed.). *Suicide.* Baltimore: Williams and Wilkins.

Sandifer MG, A Hodern, GC Timburg, and LM Green. 1968. Psychiatric diagnosis: A comparative study in North Carolina, London, and Glasgow. *Br J Psychiatry* 114: 1–9.

Sargant W. 1961. Drugs in the treatment of depression. *Br Med J* 1: 225–27.

———. 1967. *Unquiet mind: The autobiography of a physician in psychological medicine.* London: Heinemann.

Sargant W, and E Slater. 1954. *An introduction to physical methods of treatment in psychiatry,* 3rd ed. Edinburgh: E & S Livingstone. Originally published in 1944.

Saunders JC, and NS Kline. 1959. Drugs for treatment of depression. *Neurology* 9: 224–27.

Schielle BC, and WM Benson. 1960. Antidepressant medications. *Postgrad Med* 28: 101–11.

Schildkraut JJ, and SS Kety. 1967. Biogenic amine and emotion. *Science* 156: 21–30.

Schioldann JA. 2001. *The Lange theory of "periodical depressions": A landmark in the history of lithium therapy.* Adelaide: Adelaide Academic Press.

Schulberg HC, JL Coulehan, MR Block, CP Scott, SD Imber, and JM Perel. 1991. Strategies for evaluating treatments for major depression in primary care patients. *Gen Hosp Psychiatry* 13: 9–18.

Schulberg HC, MR Block, MJ Madonia, E Rodriguez, CP Scott, and J Lave. 1995. Applicability of clinical pharmacotherapy guidelines for major depression in primary care settings. *Arch Fam Med* 4: 106–12.

Schulberg HC, MR Block, MJ Madonia, CP Scott, E Rodriguez, SD Imber, et al. 1996. Treating major depression in primary care practice: Eight-month clinical outcomes. *Arch Gen Psychiatry* 53: 913–19.

Schulberg HC, MR Block, MJ Madonia, et al. 1997. The "usual care" of major depression in primary care practice. *Arch Fam Med* 6, no. 4: 334–39.

Schulberg HC, W Katon, GE Simon, and AJ Rush. 1998. Treating major depression in primary care practice: An update of the Agency for Health Care Policy and Research Practice Guidelines. *Arch Gen Psychiatry* 55: 1121–27.

Scott J, CA Moon, CV Blacker, and JM Thomas. 1994. Edinburgh Primary Care Depression Study. *Br J Psychiatry* 164: 410–415.

Scott R, JAD Anderson, and A Cartwright. 1960. Just what the doctor ordered: An analysis of treatment in a general practice. *Br Med J* ii: 293–99.

Scull A. 1989. *Social order/mental disorder: Anglo-American psychiatry in a historical perspective.* London: Routledge.

Sedgewick P. 1982. *Psychopolitics.* London: Pluts Press.

Shapiro S, PS German, EA Skinner, M VonKorff, RW Turner, LE Klein, ML Teitelbaum, M Kramer, JD Burke, and BJ Burns. 1987. An experiment to change detection and management of mental morbidity in primary care. *Med Care* 25: 327–39.

Shea MT, I Elkin, SD Imber, SM Sotsky, JT Watkins, JF Collins, PA Pilkonis, E Beckham, DR Glass, RT Dolan, et al. 1992. Course of depressive symptoms over follow-up: Findings from the National Institute of Mental Health Treatment of Depression Collaborative Research Program. *Arch Gen Psychiatry* 49: 782–87.

Sheehan JC. 1982. *The enchanted ring: The untold story of penicillin.* Cambridge: MIT Press.

Shepherd M. 1976. Foreword to *Psychiatry in dissent: Controversial issues in thought and practice* by AW Clare. London: Tavistock Publications.

———. 1977. A representative psychiatrist: The career and contributions of Sir Aubrey Lewis. *Am J Psychiatry* 134: 7–13.

Shepherd M, B Cooper, AC Brown, and GGW Kalton. 1964. Minor mental illness in London: Some aspects of a general practice survey. *Br. Med J* ii: 1359–63.

———. 1966. *Psychiatric illness in general practice.* London: Oxford University Press.

Shepherd M, G Wilkinson, and P Williams. 1986. *Mental illness in primary care settings.* London: Tavistock Publications.

Shorter E. 1985. *Bedside manners: The troubled history of doctors and patients.* New York: Viking.

———. 1997. *A history of psychiatry: From the era of the asylum to the age of prozac.* New York: John Wiley and Sons.

Shoulders HH. 1946. Medical progress in the United States under freedom: President's address. *JAMA* 131: 801–4.

Simon GE, W Katon, C Rutter, M Von Korff, E Lin, P Robinson, et al. 1998. Impact of improved depression treatment in primary care on daily functioning and disability. *Psychol Med* 28: 693–701.

Simon GE, M VonKorff, C Rutter, and E Wagner. 2000. Randomised trial of monitoring, feedback, and management of care by telephone to improve treatment of depression in primary care. *Br Med J* 320: 550–554.

Skocpol T. 1996. *Boomerang: Clinton's health security effort and the turn against government in U.S. politics.* New York: Norton.

Skrabanek, P. 1994. *The death of humane medicine and the rise of coercive healthism: The Social Affairs Unit*. Bury St. Edmunds: St. Edmundsbury Press.

Smith G. 1997. *Cambridgeshire airfields in the Second World War*. Newbury: Countryside Books.

Sobel D. 1996. *Longitude*. London: Fourth Estate.

Song F, N Freemantle, TA Sheldon, A House, P Watson, A Long, et al. 1993. Selective serotonin reuptake inhibitors: Meta-analysis of efficacy and acceptability. *Br Med J* 306: 683–87.

Spitzer RL, J Endicott, and E Robins. 1978. Research diagnostic criteria. *Arch Gen Psychiatry* 35: 773–82.

Spitzer RL, JB Williams, K Kroenke, et al. 1994. Utility of a new procedure for diagnosing mental disorders. *JAMA* 272, no. 22: 1749–56.

Srole L, TS Langner, ST Michael, MK Opler, and TAC Rennie. 1962. *Mental health in the metropolis: The Midtown Manhattan Study*. New York: McGraw-Hill.

Starfield B. 1991. Primary care and health: A cross-national comparison. *JAMA* 266, no. 16: 2268–71.

———. 1992. Primary care: Concept, evaluation, and policy. New York: Oxford University Press.

Starr P. 1982. *The social transformation of American medicine*. New York: Basic Books.

Sternbach LH. 1978. The benzodiazepine story. *Prog Drug Res* 22: 229–66.

Stevens R. 1998. *American medicine and the public interest*. Berkeley: University of California Press.

Stocks P. 1949. *Studies on medical and population subjects:* No. 2. *Sickness in the population of England and Wales, 1944–1947*. London: HMSO.

Stoeckle JD, IK Zola, and GE Davidson. 1964. The quantity and significance of psychological distress in medical patients. *J Chronic Dis* 17: 959–70.

Stone MH. 1997. *Healing the mind: A history of psychiatry from antiquity to the present*. New York: W.W. Norton.

Stunkard AJ. 1950. A method of evaluating a therapeutic agent: Results of a study of dibenamine. *Am J Psychiatry* 107: 463–67.

Styron William. 1990. *Darkness visible: A memoir of madness*. New York: Random House.

Taylor S. 1954. *Good general practice*. London: Oxford University Press.

Teasdale JD. 1999. Emotional processing, three modes of mind and the prevention of relapse in depression. *Behav Res Ther* 37: S53–S77.

Temerlin MK. 1968. Suggestion effects in psychiatric diagnosis. *J Nerv Ment Dis* 147: 349–53.

Thase ME. 1999. How should efficacy be evaluated in randomized clinical trials of treatments for depression? *J Clin Psychiatry* 60(Suppl 4): 23–31.

Thomas KB. 1978. The consultation and the therapeutic illusion. *Br Med J* i: 1327–28.

Twain M. 1906. *What is man?* New York: De Vinne Press.

Twain M. 1894. *The tragedy of Pudd'nhead Wilson*. Hartford, Conn.: American Publishing Company.

Tyrer P. 1978. Drug treatment of psychiatric patients in general practice. *Br Med J* 2: 1008–10.

Unützer J, W Katon, CM Callahan, et al. 2002. Collaborative care management improves treatment and outcomes of late life depression: A multi-site randomized trial with 1,801 depressed older adults. *JAMA* 288: 2836–45.

Ustun TB, and N. Sartorius. 1995. *Mental illness in general health care: An international study*. Chichester: John Wiley and Sons.

Verhaak PFM. 1995. *Mental disorder in the community and in general practice.* Avebury: Aldershot.

Vickers G. 1984. What sets the goals of public health? In: The Open Systems Group (eds.). *The Vickers Papers.* London: Harper and Row.

Vogel MJ, and CE Rosenberg. 1979. *The therapeutic revolution.* Philadelphia: University of Pennsylvania Press.

Von Korff M, W Katon, T Bush, EH Lin, GE Simon, et al. 1998. Treatment costs, cost offset, and cost-effectiveness of collaborative management of depression. *Psychosom Med* 60: 143–49.

Wadsworth MEJ, WJH Butterfield, and R Blaney. 1971. *Health and sickness: The choice of treatment.* London: Tavistock Publications.

Wagner EH, BT Austin, and M Von Korff. 1996. Organizing care for patients with chronic illness. *Milbank Q* 74: 511–44.

Watkin B. 1978. *The national health service: The first phase. 1948–1974 and after.* London: George Allen and Unwin.

Watts CAH, and E Stengel. 1966. *Depressive disorders in the community.* Bristol: John Wright and Sons.

Watts CAH, and BM Watts. 1952. *Psychiatry in general practice.* London: J and A Churchill.

Weatherall M. 1990. *In search of a cure: A history of pharmaceutical discovery.* Oxford: Oxford University Press.

Webster C. 1988. *The Health Services since the War:* Vol. 1. *Problems of Health Care: The National Health Service before 1957.* London: HMSO.

Weider A, K Brodman, B Mittelman, D Wechsler, and HG Wolff. 1945. Cornell Service Index: A method for quickly assaying personality and psychosomatic disturbances among men in the armed forces. *War-Med* 7: 209–13.

———. 1946. The Cornell Index: A method for quickly assaying personality and psychosomatic disturbances, to be used as an adjunct to interview. *Psychosom Med* 8: 411–13.

Weissman MM, and GL Klerman. 1977. The chronic depressives in the community: Unrecognized and poorly treated. *Compr Psychiatry* 18: 523–32.

Wells KB, A Stewart, RD Hays, et al. 1989. The functioning and well-being of depressed patients. *JAMA* 262, no. 7: 914–19.

Wells KB, C Sherbourne, M Schoenbaum, N Duan, L Meredith, J Unützer, J Miranda, MF Carney, and LV Rubenstein. 2000. Impact of disseminating quality improvement programs for depression in managed primary care: A randomized controlled trial. *JAMA* 283: 212–20.

Wheatley D. 1969. A comparative trial of imipramine and phenobarbital in depressed patients seen in general practice. *J Nerv Ment Dis* 148: 542–49.

———. 1972. Evaluation of psychotropic drugs in general practice. *Proc R Soc Med* 65: 317–20.

White KL, TF Williams, and BG Greenberg. 1961. The ecology of medical care. *N Engl J Med* 265: 885–92.

WHO Collaborating Centre for Mental Health Research and Training. 2000. *WHO guide to mental health in primary care.* London: Institute of Psychiatry.

Wilbanks E. 1972. The doctor as romantic hero: A study of idealization. *JAMA* 220: 54–57.

Wilkinson RG. 1992. National mortality rates: The impact of inequality? *Am J Public Health* 82, no. 8: 1082–84.

———. 1999. Income inequality, social cohesion, and health: Clarifying the theory. *Int J Health Serv* 29, no. 3: 525–43.

Williams TI. 1984. *Howard Florey: Penicillin and after.* Oxford: Oxford University Press.

Williamson J. 1964. Old people at home: Their unreported needs. *Lancet* I: 1117–19.

Wilson M. 1993. DSM-III and the transformation of American psychiatry: A history. *Am J Psychiatry* 150: 339–410.

Wilson S. 1995. *Tate Gallery: An illustrated companion.* London: Tate Gallery Publishing.

Wing JK, JE Cooper, and N Sartorius. 1974. *The description and classification of psychiatric symptoms: An instruction manual for the PSE and CATEGO system.* London: Cambridge University Press.

Wing JK, P Bebbington, and LN Robins. 1981. *What is a case? The problem of definition in psychiatric community surveys.* London: Grant McIntyre.

Woods JW, JD Dorsett, KL White, H Smith, R Hill, and J Watson. 1958. The evaluation of "medical" therapy in essential hypertension. *J Psychosom Res* 2: 274–84.

Working Group on First-Contact Mental Health Care. 1984. *First-contact mental health care: Report on a WHO meeting, Tampere, Finland, 25–29 April 1983.* Albany, NY: WHO Publications Center USA.

World Health Organization. 1978. *Alma Alta 1978: Primary health care: Report of the International Conference on Primary Health Care.* Geneva: World Health Organization.

_____. 2001. *World health report 2001, mental health: New understanding, new hope.* Geneva: World Health Organization.

Zubin J. 1954. Presidential address: Biometric methods in psychopathology. In: PE Hoch and J Zubin (eds.). *Depression.* Oxford: Grune and Stratton.

Zung WWK, and King RE. 1983. Identification and treatment of masked depression in a general medical practice. *J Clin Psychiatry* 44: 365–68.

Index

Italic page numbers indicate illustrations and graphics.